Gustavo Sánchez

A Rebel Unconscious

Interrogating the Desire for Social Change in Chile's Estallido

palgrave
macmillan

Gustavo Sánchez
Institute of Psychiatry, Psychology &
Neuroscience
King's College London
London, UK

ISSN 2662-2629 ISSN 2662-2637 (electronic)
Studies in the Psychosocial
ISBN 978-3-032-12274-2 ISBN 978-3-032-12275-9 (eBook)
https://doi.org/10.1007/978-3-032-12275-9

Cover credit: Vladimir Lis

This Palgrave Macmillan imprint is published by the registered company Springer Nature Switzerland AG
The registered company address is: Gewerbestrasse 11, 6330 Cham, Switzerland

To my mum, Lucila, who's gold enough.

Acknowledgments Probably since its inception, I rejected the idea that this book was about me. Some well-intended yet, in my view, extreme versions of positionality in the current research atmosphere do not sit well with me. I always assumed that people suggesting such a parallel were trying to put me into that box: you are Chilean and critical, so this *must* be about you. When the final month to submit the manuscript arrived, I had morbid intrusive thoughts that led to paralysing anxiety. After seven years, I went back to analysis. In my initial session, during the introduction, my analyst said the same thing: so your research is about yourself. I think I reacted graciously, but I did not like that. My anxiety was horrendous and that same day I saw one of my closest friends—who happens to be one of the most amazing humans and a talented psychoanalyst—for a chat. When I told her about my exasperation with the idea that I was writing about myself, all she had to do was roll her eyes. That was when the penny finally dropped, and I realised that this book is about me in the most substantial way: not because I am Chilean, or an academic, or have been affected by the revolt, but because the mere idea of change paralyses me. I would rather imagine and try to convince myself that I am the worst than accept that I can be different. In that sense, I am no different from the people I interviewed and observed for this book. On a more personal note, I am thankful to all of them for granting me the psychically painful realisation of that.

Many people offered me their kindness and support during the years this project took place. Karla Bray, Liza van Munsteren, and Stacey Clapperton got the lion's share—and I hope I can do justice, in whatever form, to their immense love. Vincent Harting and Bruno Lloret became brothers by destiny, with all the beautiful familial insecurities. Daniel Leyton and Francisca Jalil looked after me when I needed it most, asking nothing in return. Stephen Frosh and Margarita Palacios walked me through the, at times, terrifying doctoral training. A brief yet generous encounter with Todd McGowan gave me the reassurance to conclude this book when the path looked daunting. Pancho, Andrea, Julia, Coté, Sebastián, Lucas, Víctor, María Luisa, Irina, and Felipe were all in Chile but never too far. If there are any good lines in this book, it is because my family—especially my mum and my brothers—have taught me all the important things I know. And one day I was lucky enough to bump into Layla Orr; since then, there has been no day short on magic—or change.

London, September 2025

Competing Interests This work was supported by the Agencia Nacional de Investigación y Desarrollo (Becas Chile No. 72200242).

Ethics Approval The Ethics Committee of the School of Social Sciences, History and Philosophy at Birkbeck, University of London, granted the author approval to conduct the fieldwork for his research on 7 March 2022.

Contents

About the Author

Gustavo Sánchez holds a PhD in Psychosocial Studies from Birkbeck, University of London, and is a Qualitative Research Associate in the Institute of Psychiatry, Psychology & Neuroscience at King's College London.

1

Social Change Is Hard (to Understand)

The *Estallido*: Between Restoration and Power

For the past three decades, scholars and commentators in the West have deemed neoliberalism one of the main obstacles to a good life. Despite the standard Anglophone narrative that locates the political rise of neoliberalism in Thatcher and Reagan, it is well-established that Chile became a crash test dummy for experimenting with this set of policies in the 1970s, earning the unglamorous title of the 'laboratory' of neoliberalism (Barder, 2013). Along with the rampant inequality sparked off by privatisation, marketisation, and deregulation (Cahill, 2014), neolib eralism has been depicted as the expansion of competition into the ruling mindset of our times, encouraging all sorts of excessive practices (Dardot & Laval, 2017). Rather unsurprisingly, then, neoliberal policies have stirred popular indignation over the unfulfilled promises of betterment that market expansion allegedly once held (Almeida & Pérez, 2022). 'Malaise' is the term most interpretations of this indignation coalesced around in Chile (Atria et al., 2014; Brunner, 1998; Moyano, 2021; Ruiz & Boccardo, 2015; Vera, 2017). The prominence of this idea simultaneously provides a window into the country's recent past

G. Sánchez, *A Rebel Unconscious*, Studies in the Psychosocial,
https://doi.org/10.1007/978-3-032-12275-9_1

and the workings of social change. Literally 'bad-ease', malaise points to the discomfort provoked by a diffuse agent that, from the outside, impedes our comfort. Getting rid of the neoliberal obstacle, following this logic, would allow us to sit comfortably, to experience 'good-ease' so to speak.

At least since 2006, successive popular mobilisations have sought to fight back against the neoliberal-induced discomfort in Chile. Secondary and higher education, pensions, the environment, and gender are some of the areas where neoliberal policies have been challenged over the past twenty years (Rodríguez, 2020). These relatively regional struggles are the direct antecedents of Chile's revolt in 2019. During the concluding months of that year, a series of seemingly isolated student protests against the increase in tube fares led to what many consider the largest popular uprising in Chile's history (Castillo, 2019; Landaeta & Herrero, 2021; Martuccelli, 2019; Ruiz, 2020). Unlike previous demonstrations, the tone and nature of the protests were markedly distinct: rather than demanding the improvement of a circumscribed aspect of society, the revolt staged a visceral rejection of the prevailing organisation of life, acquiring an existential condition (Villalobos-Ruminott, 2020). The *estallido* ('outburst'), as the uprising is popularly known, turned Chile into an almost unrecognisable place shaped by a collective desire for social change that heralded a post-neoliberal era. Between 18 October and 31 December 2019, over 3,000 protest actions of varying scale took place in Chile (Somma et al., 2020). On 25 October, in Santiago alone, more than a million people joined what is widely considered the largest demonstration in Chilean history—in a country whose population at the time was around 19 million. After decades of sitting uncomfortably, Chileans suddenly found themselves not merely resisting the neoliberal obstacle to a good life but actually removing it.

The above is far from a hyperbolic statement. In the view of Sebastián Edwards (2019)—UCLA professor, former Chief Economist for Latin America at the World Bank, and neoliberal enthusiast—one of the few things that became clear after the *estallido* was that 'the neoliberal experiment is dead'. By admission of its very supporters, we were stepping into something different. Accordingly, it is no surprise that, from progressive academia, the revolt was portrayed as 'the end of the neoliberal consensus' (Ferretti & Dragnic, 2020, p. 123), 'the end of the Chilean way to neoliberalism' (Cortés, 2022, p. 90) or, even more directly, 'the experience of the end of neoliberalism' (Castillo, 2019, p. 42).[1] For the first time since the neoliberal modernisation unfurled, an unobstructed life seemed within reach for the Chilean people. My claim is that, despite the vast body of literature on the *estallido*, the experience it brought about remains understudied. As a result of the entrenchment of certain analytical premises, scholarship swears by the idea that in the absence of external obstacles, nothing would stand between us and social change. In other words, without the deception of ideological machinations and the coercion of power inequality, embracing socially desirable goals—such as a post-neoliberal society—should be a no-brainer. The Chilean revolt presents an opportunity to interrogate the validity of the traditional paradigm of social change and the limitations of dominant frameworks for its study. These are, respectively, the restorative approach and power-centred models.

Let us begin with how social change is assumed to operate. In many respects, the way we conceive of it harks back to Marx and his critique of capitalist alienation as a force that separates us from nature. In the *Economic and Philosophic Manuscripts of 1844*, he famously linked private property to the worker's alienated or estranged labour and distilled three of its manifestations: alienation in the product of labour (this product exists outside and independently from the worker), alienation in the labour process (in forced labour the worker denies themselves), and the alienation of universality (the worker is separated from nature, the means of their life, and instrument of their life-activity). Consequently, Marx (1978, p. 84) defined communism as a way of countering alienation: '*Communism* as the *positive* transcendence of *private property*, or *human self-estrangement*, and therefore as the real *appropriation of the human* essence by and for man; communism therefore as the complete return of man to himself as a *social* (i.e., human) being'. The idea that alienation is both contingent and problematic paved the way for a restorative conceptualisation of social change: we should rebel against

[1] All direct quotations from Spanish sources—including fieldwork material—have been translated by the author.

human self-estrangement *to regain access* to an original or primeval state. In this vein, social change becomes an emancipatory impulse to collectively remove whatever external obstacle prevents us from being who we truly are.

Despite widespread backlash against essentialism in contemporary critical theory, the *estallido* has nonetheless been subjected to restorative analyses. One of the clearest ways in which this occurs is through its portrayal as a suspension of symbolic mediation in favour of the presumed anarchic potency of bodies impounded by neoliberalism. From this perspective, by way of example, the *estallido* is perceived as a 'destituent potency' manifesting as an 'instant communism' (Galende, 2020, p. 55). This movement does not challenge the order of things through an alternative discourse but rather through a 'bodily potency' that operates as a law unto itself—'it is born of itself and is not subordinated to any text or script that explains it' (p. 54). A similar interpretation can be found in the idea of the 'mythical immediacy' of the *estallido* proposed by Willy Thayer (2023, p. 849), a process 'established and exercised based on its own jurisdiction and authority, and in antagonism to Chile's neoliberal design'. These restorative approaches locate the emancipatory character of the revolt in its capacity to overcome alienation through the radical disorganisation of our neoliberal world (see also Karmy, 2019, 2020).

Let us now turn to how social change is customarily studied. For reasons that may seem self-evident, power relations have long been central to this field of enquiry. In his insightful examination of the logics of political organisation, Rodrigo Nunes (2021) fleshes out the centrality of power by drawing on Baruch Spinoza's distinction between *potestas* and *potentia*. In a world broadly divided between the powerful and the weak, the former have what Spinoza terms *potestas*, namely, an array of tangible and intangible resources they can wield to ensure their will prevails. The weak, by contrast, lack *potestas*; their only asset is their capacity to act. This is *potentia*, the ability to affect and be affected by others. In isolation, *potentia* is insufficient to counter *potestas*, yet through mutual affectation a collective subject can emerge to transform the existing conditions. Much of the scholarship on social change takes some variation of this framework as its epistemological foundation.

In one way or another, the point is to understand how the powerful acquire and sustain their power and how the weak might overcome their subjugation to effect change.

Many variations of the power-centred models have been applied to the *estallido*. A widely accepted narrative regarding the causes of the revolt emphasises the cumulative effect of successive social movements over the past decade in Chile. According to the historian Luis Thielemann (2020), the revolt represents the culmination of a cycle that began in 2011. That year, young students from working and middle-class backgrounds forged an alliance rooted in a critique of the neoliberal order and the unfulfilled promises of social mobility. Such an alliance marked a significant expansion, both quantitative and qualitative, of popular resistance to neoliberalism in the country, later expressed through mobilisations against the pension system and the feminist movement (Asún et al., 2020). Along similar lines, Pierre Dardot (2023) interprets the *estallido* as the product of a series of social movements that engendered various 'collective subjectivations' in opposition to what he terms 'the experience of neoliberalism' in Chile. For Dardot, a proper understanding of the revolt requires examining how different actors contributed to shaping political commitments against concrete, everyday manifestations of neoliberalism. In this sense, the historical struggle for social, political, and cultural recognition of indigenous peoples, alongside the renewed prominence of the feminist movement from the mid-2010s onwards, can be seen as part of the political subjectivations that enabled the *estallido* to challenge the neoliberal *potestas*.

A Psychoanalytic Account of Emancipatory Identifications

For most scholars, the Chilean revolt has been—and likely continues to be—regarded as a validation of the analytical premises buttressing much of the literature on social change: the eradication of alienation as its ultimate goal and power as its essential analytical unit. This book argues, however, that the *estallido* calls these premises into question. I advance a psychoanalytic interpretation of the revolt's experience that demonstrates the unfitness of the restorative approach and the insufficiency of power-based models in understanding the experience of social change. At its most basic, accepting the existence of the psychoanalytic unconscious implies locating disharmony (or alienation) at the centre of our experience of the world and of ourselves. This means that we are not only *accidentally* or *historically* prevented from experiencing good-ease due to oppressive power relations; more fundamentally, we are *constitutively* incapable of overcoming a baseline level of disharmony. If we were to believe psychoanalysis, we should therefore be cautious about attempts to do away with alienation and to make power the overriding explanatory principle of our experience. In contrast, I argue for the necessity of incorporating an account of unconscious desire into the study of social change.

Owing to its overwhelming emphasis on power, the literature on social change tends to gloss over psychoanalytic theory. Take one of the most recent treatises on the subject. Richard Ballard and Clive Barnett (2023) edited *The Routledge Handbook of Social Change*, a 400-page volume with contributions from 32 experts in the field. The editors acknowledge that no handbook can provide a comprehensive overview of social change, though it can offer selective entry points for future developments. However diverse these entry points may be, they follow a notably uniform pattern: the term 'power' appears over 400 times in the book, while 'unconscious' only once—and in a non-technical fashion. The message is indirect yet unmistakable: power is the default entry point to study social change and the latter is none of psychoanalysis' business. The dominance of power-centred models has undoubtedly sharpened our awareness of strategies, positions, and forms of resistance. Yet such frameworks remain ill-equipped to grasp the lived experience of an event like the *estallido*. By this I mean the process of forging a commitment to a different organisation of life that, while reasonably *deduced* from the effects of the unequal distribution of power, cannot be wholly *reduced* to these power relations. As the incisive analysis of Joan Copjec (2015) demonstrated long ago, the assumption that society is nothing more than the sum of its internal networks of power and knowledge relations necessarily avoids the question of desire.

In all fairness, psychoanalysis itself has also contributed to evading the question of desire in social change research. With a handful of notable exceptions (Kapoor, 2020; Kornbluh, 2022; McGowan, 2022; Ruti, 2018), psychoanalytic approaches have tacitly accepted that they have little to say about the production of progressive political commitments. One could argue that the most innovative application of psychoanalysis in social research lies in the exploration of unconscious dynamics to deepen the critique of ideology (Daly, 1999; Glynos, 2001). Over the past two decades, particularly Lacanian notions such as enjoyment, fantasy, and desire have been successfully employed to study the clandestine side of discourses and the ways they secure identification through the production of desiring narratives (e.g., Bloom, 2016; Hoedemaekers, 2019; Hook, 2020; Palacios, 2011; Sánchez et al., 2024). Focusing scholarly attention on the unconscious dynamics underpinning retrograde or oppressive practices is undoubtedly valuable in the face of increasingly subtle forms of domination. Yet somehow, limiting psychoanalysis to the exploration of such phenomena makes it seem unnecessary to be equally attentive to progressive identifications, thereby strengthening the perception that the desire for social change encounters only external obstacles.

My book seeks to demonstrate the benefits of psychoanalysis for studying emancipatory identifications. In her study of the psychic toll of working for social change, Hannah Proctor (2024, p. 59) dwells on Ranajit Guha's remark about the 'rebel consciousness' of peasants during the Indian colonial period and leaves a question hanging in the air: 'Would it also be possible to talk about something like a rebel unconscious?'. If I filched this formulation for the title of my book, it is because it neatly encapsulates the dialectic at play in the *estallido*: far from assuming the unconscious as a site of creative, rebellious potency (e.g., Berardi, 2021), the rebelliousness of the unconscious stems from its capacity to destabilise our conscious attempts to rebel against social oppression.[2] The wager of my book is that the desire for social

[2] For Lacanian psychoanalysis, desire is primarily related to the Other and not to the object; it is the result of our uprooting from the field of necessity effectuated by the symbolic. This is why 'desire presents itself as what, in the demand for love, *rebels against being reduced to a need*, because in reality it satisfies nothing other than itself, that is, desire as an absolute condition'

change leads not to the confirmation of who we are but to an experience of alienation. As Yannis Stavrakakis (2019, p. 5) puts it, the unconscious is 'a *hypothesis* based on a series of troubling phenomena that otherwise remain obscure and inexplicable'. My empirical study of identifications with the *estallido* examines several instances in which individuals go to extraordinary lengths to sustain the desirable experience of having removed the neoliberal obstacle. Without the hypothesis of a rebel unconscious, it would be impossible to explain why it is so hard to accept that we can now sit more comfortably.

It is important to state that my exploration is rooted in a particular tradition and does not aspire to speak on behalf of the entire psychoanalytic field. I draw from two related sources. First, the scholarship that, since the 1990s, has made sustained efforts to underscore the relevance of Lacanian theory for the study of social and cultural phenomena, broadly understood (Glynos & Stavrakakis, 2008; Ruti, 2012; Žižek, 1997). Mark Bracher's *Lacan, Discourse, and Social Change* stands as a key inspiration for my own project. Already in the early 1990s, he challenged mainstream approaches to cultural studies by linking social change to desire rather than power. His Lacanian approach to interpellation led him to focus on problems around identification in standard discourse theory, such as the precise elements of a discourse that promote identification, the psychic structures involved in this process, and how change manifests in those who engage in identification. Overall, his conceptualisation of the unconscious dynamics at play in eliciting or resisting change suggests that identification should be understood as a mode of desire and, consequently, as a conflictual dynamic: 'when an identification becomes established as our identity, it functions to repress all desires that are incongruent with this identity' (Bracher, 1993, p. 22).

The second source is the more recent set of attempts to delineate Lacanian methodological principles for empirical research, such as Lacanian Discourse Analysis (LDA) (Bucci et al., 2022; Hook, 2013; Neill, 2013) and Critical Fantasy Studies (CFS) (Glynos, 2021; Glynos et al., 2019; Ronderos & Glynos, 2022). What differentiates these approaches is their

(Lacan, 2017, p. 362, emphasis added). In any desire, including the desire for social change, being loved by the Other is unconsciously much more important than getting the object.

emphasis on specific periods of Lacanian epistemology. Researchers affiliated with LDA take as their overriding premise the non-rapport of the structural positions of a given discourse, a perspective developed in the later stage of Lacan's teaching. Discourses can be understood as particular ways of addressing the absence of a social bond. Researchers therefore aim to identify which structural position takes the reins of the master signifier in each case, concealing this impossibility. Studies following the coordinates of CFS grant greater importance to subjective overinvestment in ideology, usually channelled through fantasies, and draw on earlier periods of Lacan's work. As Jason Glynos maintains: 'the idea of resistance to change, or its opposite, rapid transformation, are very abstract problem domains that I think the notions of fantasy and enjoyment can help shed light on, making clear their relevance to questions of ideology' (Glynos et al., 2019, p. 149). In both cases, the unconscious is operationalised as a property of symbolic production—i.e., the fact that human action is always mediated by language—rather than as a psychological feature of the individual. This brings the Lacanian unconscious closer to the psychosocial project of bridging the social and the psychic dimensions of our experience (Frosh et al., 2024; Lapping, 2011).

Furthermore, I turn to the Lacanian tradition in a selective fashion. My study draws on a defined set of key technical terms, which I will elaborate on in Chapter 2: desire, fantasy, Other, imaginary, symbolic, and unconscious. These concepts provide me with the essential elements to conduct an exploration of the libidinal economy of the *estallido*. Whenever this flamboyant concept appears in this book, it should be understood as a particular type of organisation: the organisation of our psychic life. And these key terms are necessary because our psychic life is notoriously arduous to organise. More precisely, libidinal economy captures the unconscious circuits of *excess* and *antagonism* that accompany our conscious practices; in this case, the conscious commitment to social change (see Kapoor et al., 2023; Kapoor, 2020). Our psychic life is hard to organise—or, even better, we find it hard to understand and tolerate its organisation—because our desires 'obey a logic that runs counter to reason and predictability, often diverting and undermining intentions, plans, and projects' (Kapoor et al., 2023, p. 8). From a Lacanian perspective, the study of the desire for social change brings to the fore *the structural alienation* of the subject and the ensuing impossibility of achieving full sovereignty in its pursuits, however laudable they may be.

Since my objective is to show that there is a dimension of the experience of social change not captured by dominant approaches, I strategically focused my study on a specific group of people: critical scholars. My primary interest lies in the position they occupy within the social division of labour—they are likely the only group for whom social change is a professional occupation. In other words, society acknowledges their intellectual commitment to social change and positions them as experts on the matter—their commitment is both socially and self-recognised. Given this dual recognition, it is warranted to assume that their identification with social change is far less problematic than that of others. If the restorative approach is correct, then an emancipatory event like the *estallido* must have been akin to a moment of plenitude for critical scholars. Conversely, if I can demonstrate that *even* their identifications with the *estallido* were shaped by unconscious excess and antagonism, this would evince that alienation is part and parcel of emancipatory experiences as such.

I adopt here the rationale of critical case sampling (Patton, 2002, p. 263), which involves selecting a case based on its significance for establishing logical generalisations following the premise that 'if it happens here, it will happen anywhere'. Consequently, if someone who consciously embraces social change still unconsciously struggles to identify with the *estallido*, it is reasonable to infer that this is a general experience. My decision is thus methodological rather than political. I do not suggest that critical academics are better equipped to address social change, closer to the revolution than other groups, or the sole embodiment of 'critical' subjectivity. Rather, since they 'promote the emancipation from exploitation, oppression and exclusion' (Loick, 2018, p. 233), their subjectivities are consciously, ordinarily, and intimately shaped by social change (I will conceptualise this in Chapter 2). In sum, I have not chosen critical scholars because they are the best rebels out there, but because they are in a particularly advantageous position to grasp the rebelliousness of the unconscious in the process of identifying with emancipatory events. I follow here a simple maxim: 'even the most politically committed individuals have contradictory psychic lives that can impede or complicate their political activities' (Proctor, 2024, p. 6).

With the above in mind, I spent four months in Chile during the first half of 2022 conducting individual interviews with scholars and PhD researchers, as well as observing three doctoral modules (see Appendix). I produced my material—28 interviews and over 40 hours of observations—following the principle of free association described by Freud. That is, I asked my interviewees to keep an idea in mind as a starting point (the *estallido*) and follow whatever path this idea led them down. For the observations, my field notes traced the use of the word '*estallido*' and its further associations. This symbolic account frames the unconscious not as 'our own private secret but what we constantly demonstrate to others through our speech and acts' (McGowan, 2024, p. 17). The next chapter will expand on my interpretive strategy. Meanwhile, I should flag up that the associations elicited by the term '*estallido*' revealed the complex psychic organisation of this event at an unconscious level, conspicuously expressed in the difficulties these subjects faced in retaining a sense of coherence in their identification with the revolt. It turns out that the call inviting them to identify with the *estallido* was full of gaps that they had to fill through imaginary narratives or fantasies. My analysis focused on reconstructing some of these fantasies.

The Trauma of Removing Cherished Obstacles

I have taken this alternative route to studying the experience of social change because Lacanian psychoanalysis suggests an outrageous hypothesis: what if we must protect ourselves from getting what we want? Or, to put it differently, what if achieving social change is a traumatic experience? A simple way to illustrate this idea is by reflecting on the main motto of the *estallido*: Chile woke up. This rallying cry became so popular partly because it succinctly conveyed that neoliberalism forced us to live an unacceptable life, and now we could finally see clearly that change was imperative. While this is undeniable, the emphasis on its social undesirability should not make us lose sight of the fact that, quite literally, *neoliberalism was forcing us to live* (a socially unacceptable life). And altering what makes us alive, even if we do not like the way we are living, is psychically hard to endure. The lesson here is that the psychic life of objects does not follow the same logic as the social realm. Two people may acknowledge the perniciousness of neoliberalism—say, in terms of the erosion of a sense of community in their neighbourhoods—yet while one of them might have seen in the *estallido* a way of rebelling against this, the other might refrain from engagement. This is not because the second person suddenly finds neoliberalism agreeable, but, as Alenka Zupančič (2000, pp. 34–5) puts it, 'because the object at stake does not play the same part in the libidinal economy of the two people'.

Given the above, psychoanalysis begins by acknowledging that a conscious obstacle can have an entirely different value for our unconscious life. That is why we often have to fight against ourselves to commit to healthier lifestyles, early nights, nutritious diets… and emancipatory events. There is a complex and profoundly ambivalent unconscious organisation of our identifications that creates psychic conflicts in the pursuit of consciously desirable goals. Regardless of how damaging certain obstacles to a good life may be, we often come to cherish them because they negatively constitute us—and this is always preferable to not being constituted at all. For Adam Phillips (2018, p. 34) symptoms 'are always construed by the patient as obstacles; so it is always worth wondering what the patient's imaginary unobstructed life would look like in the absence of such constraints'. Furthermore, he maintains that symptoms are 'cherished obstacles' that stage counterintuitive scenarios marked by catastrophe and pleasure. Adapting this idea to my purpose here, studying the fantasies that structure the desire for social change in the *estallido* offers us a glimpse into what our imaginary unobstructed life looks like in the absence of the cherished obstacle called neoliberalism. From this perspective, the sociological existence of neoliberalism is only part of the problem. Even in a world where entrepreneurial mindsets were rejected, competition gave way to collaboration, and private property ceased to exist, we would still have to reckon with the psychic life of these obstacles.

Despite appearances, my approach differs significantly from studies of the neoliberal subjectivity based on the logic of governmentality (e.g.,

Bröckling, 2015; Dardot & Laval, 2017). These are some of the most intricate enquiries into how neoliberalism, far from simplistic portrayals of laissez-faire and state withdrawal, actively produces subjectivities. Two key features characterise these kinds of studies. On the one hand, neoliberalism can be understood as an anthropological project that seeks to turn the figure of the enterprise into the most complete way of governing human life. On the other hand, neoliberalism is an innovative regime insofar as it governs by promoting self-governing techniques. This makes neoliberalism not only a totalising discourse that aims to capture every aspect of our experience, but also an exceptionally efficient one. When it comes to social change, the conclusion here is that while overcoming neoliberalism remains possible, it is difficult to achieve because it functions all too well. My claim is precisely the opposite: there is no identification that does not hobble, so they all come with unconscious crutches. I extend this insight to argue that even when we experience the end of neoliberalism—even when we come to identify with what we consciously want—our identifications inevitably malfunction due to structural alienation. To perceive this, it is necessary to shift our focus from neoliberalism as a technology of the self to neoliberalism as the signifier that organises our psychic life.

It should now be clear why a project like this requires both breaking away from the restorative approach and softening the gravitational pull of power-centred models. In the first case, the exploration of the productive side of alienation is curtailed by the conflation of its contingent and structural manifestations. Within power-centred models, in turn, there is no room for studying neoliberalism as a cherished obstacle, that is, as a consciously damaging experience that can nonetheless provide unconscious satisfaction. Yet, in order to conduct my research, I additionally had to avoid one of the major pitfalls of my own field. With dismaying consistency, psychoanalytically inspired scholarship resorts to Lacanian theory to parrot formulaic statements that, once uttered, leave us exactly where we started. If I want to flaunt my radical Lacanian credentials, all I need to do is claim that the *estallido* was a manifestation of the return of the repressed, the unsymbolisable real in the neoliberal narrative, or invoke the capitalist discourse. This is one of the reasons behind my leaning towards notions such as imaginary, fantasy, and desire over those of the real, drive, or *jouissance*.[3] Not only am I convinced of their heuristic potential for studying the experience of social change, but they also enable the deployment of Lacanian theory to explore a phenomenon rather than taming it with oven-ready explanations.

Furthermore, the concepts underpinning my exploration of the libidinal economy of the *estallido* open up a mode of interpretation that runs counter to deep-seated academic beliefs. In a move seemingly triggered by the rejection of organisation as the source of domination and oppression (Nunes, 2021), emancipatory events tend to be portrayed and studied under the assumption that their defining feature is the undoing of all kinds of organisation. In recent years, this has taken the form of a renewed interest in the potential of imagination and speculation. The central idea here is that 'images emerge before language and contain a surplus of meaning that cannot often be rendered through linguistic descriptions' (Bottici, 2014, p. 6). This has prompted creative elaborations around the idea of the 'political imagination' as a way of moving beyond the constraints of what has historically been defined as possible and real, in order to challenge conformity (Duncombe & Harrebye, 2022; see also Browne & Diehl, 2019). At the same time, however, the primacy granted to images over the symbolic has strengthened the perception of emancipation as rupture, destabilisation, and the absence of organisation. As long as organisation is resisted, it is assumed that we are experiencing emancipation.

Let me provide one of many possible examples. Christopher Castiglia (2017a, 2017b) has explored the potential of imagination by suggesting that this faculty possesses a twofold capacity: by shaping ideals into worlds, imagination reaffirms our engagement with the social; at the same time, it renders the social an unreal possibility, allowing it to become re-imaginable. Imagination is a way of refusing the shape of our current world by extracting the element within it that has not yet been realised—it is the speculative capacity to unlock affective states that remain dormant within the current organisation of the social. This is why

[3] For a sharp examination of the trivialities to which the notion of *jouissance* can lead, see Leader, 2021.

something like hope exists for Castiglia. The key aspect of his formulation is that hope functions as a kind of autonomous process, which can have progressive effects only insofar as it keeps the social at arm's length: 'Hope attached to a specific object–a hope *for*–becomes *want*, a surrender of the self-perpetuating drive toward betterment in favor of a rearrangement of already-existing conditions' (Castiglia, 2017a, p. 222). As we can see, imagination is transformative when it is not organised or, put differently, organisation amounts to the annulment of imagination.

One of the main risks posed by the scholarly tendency that Castiglia represents is the establishment of a bar for assessing emancipatory events that no revolt or political movement could ever meet (Sánchez, 2025). Transformation is thereby reduced to the speculative affects that arise from the undoing and disorganisation of the given, and it comes to a halt as soon as we aspire to rearrange already-existing conditions. The problem is that when we conceive of change as fundamentally resisting organisation, it ceases to be *social* change. For this influential branch of political imagination, sustaining the impracticable ideal of transformation purged of impurities seems more appealing than improving life in this world. This is patently at odds with the modern tradition of transformative knowledge, at least from Marx onwards. Communism, arguably the richest concept of social change, was for Marx and Engels neither an ideal nor a singular event; it was the material movement towards the abolition of the current state of things in order to achieve a classless society (Marx & Engels, 1998)—not simply for the sake of abolishing things. This is why something like communism can only be produced 'against the grain of capitalism, alongside it and not after it' (Ross, 2024, p. 91). Social change is always a spurious or, to be more precise, an internally divided experience.

I approached the *estallido* not as the disorganisation of the neoliberal form of life in Chile but *as the organisation of a post-neoliberal experience*. Based on my cursory discussion of the political imagination, there is a world of difference between these two positions. The Spanish translation of *Proletarian Nights* includes an illuminating interview with Jacques Rancière in which he delves into the nature of his research. When revisiting the ways in which the artisans he studied distanced themselves from the system of domination they lived under, he suggests that the challenge for present-day struggles is structurally the same. This is because there is a fundamental tension in any attempt to defy domination, which is much more complex than merely retrieving the desire for emancipation from the webs of domination: 'Emancipation is a way of living inequality according to the logic of equality' (Rancière, 2010, p. 11). Adapting this formula to my study, we do not have to imagine a moment of complete transcendence of neoliberalism to deem the *estallido* emancipatory. As an impure and internally divided organisation of the social, the revolt allowed Chileans to experience neoliberalism according to the logic of post-neoliberalism. As I will show in greater detail in the next chapter, this was a symbolic process that replicated its internal division in the subject, producing circuits of unconscious excess and antagonism in the efforts to identify with the revolt.

The *estallido* was at once a unique emancipatory event and one among many anti-neoliberal mass protests of the past decade. Indeed, Vincent Bevins (2023) suggests that the 2010s were defined by a global wave of contention beginning in Tunisia in 2010 and including—among others—Egypt in 2011, Brazil and Turkey in 2013, and Lebanon, Hong Kong, and Chile in 2019. For him, the scale and intensity of these revolts makes them the largest cycle of mass protests in history. His comparative perspective highlights an intriguing aspect of the explanations offered by pundits and academics:

> After a mass protest event, social scientists and journalists begin to look for structural explanations. That country has a lot of inequality, they may say. Unemployment was high; the price of food has risen; democratic reforms are needed. All of that is hugely helpful and part of the story. But I think that after taking an extremely wide view of the decade, looking at these events in comparison to one another makes it clear that this isn't quite enough. Employing just those methods, you can't really explain why Chile's uprising happened in 2019 instead of 2015, or why Brazil had one at all. (Bevins, 2023, p. 274)

Regardless of how detailed the list of neoliberal-induced issues may be, this line of argument inevitably misses the mark. Such analyses fall prey to the historicist fallacy that, as Louis Althusser (2020) would have put it, by accounting for the aqueducts you can explain a pint of water.[4] I take this limitation as an expression of the contingency and internal division of the *estallido*. So, Bevins' observation hit the nail on the head: there is something about social change that does not quite fit. Just as we cannot unequivocally explain why the *estallido* happened despite having compelling reasons, when it did take place, we could not unambiguously find ourselves in this emancipatory event despite wanting it. This substantiates the hypothesis of a rebel unconscious—there may be something inherently traumatic about identifying with social change. In his analysis of the logics of political action, Nunes (2021) mentions in passing 'the traumas of organisation'. He refers to the fact that organisation is at once a remedy and an affliction; something one can never have in the right dose. With a slight shift in the terms of this shrewd formulation, it could be said that the goal of my enterprise is to account for the psychic organisation of the traumas of identifying with social change.

Let me schematically recapitulate my argument. Social change has been predominantly conceptualised as a process aimed at restoring our relationship to the world by removing an alienating obstacle. This premise has privileged power-centred models for the study of social change. Lacanian psychoanalysis offers a different perspective on the role that alienation plays in our identifications, but this approach has not yet been systematically deployed for the empirical study of emancipatory events. The experience of the end of neoliberalism, brought about by the Chilean revolt, serves as an opportunity to interrogate the validity of the restorative approach and the hegemony of power-centred models. Empirically studying the identification of critical academics with this event functions as a methodological strategy to highlight the role of unconscious excess and antagonism precisely where we would least expect to find them. This is what *A Rebel Unconscious* offers the reader. Once again, Adam Phillips (2021, p. 5) encapsulates exactly what drives my curiosity to engage in a study like this: 'We are the only animals for

[4] 'For no more than we can explain the water in this glass with reference to all the waterways in the world can we explain a historical fact (in the sense of an immediate historical fact) by the succession, however long and multifaceted it may be, of all the historical facts in the world' (Althusser, 2020, p. 42).

whom radical change can be an object of desire. And we are traditionally at our most ambivalent about objects of desire'. The scholarship on social change typically stops at the period; my study tries to capture the consequences of what comes after.

Structure and Content of the Chapters

The next chapters are organised as follows. Chapter 2 provides the conceptual definitions of the main terms of my study, along with my interpretive approach. I define the *estallido* as a paradoxical event—simultaneously rooted in neoliberalism yet irreducible to it—that organised a post-neoliberal experience. Rather than offering an opportunity to imagine what a post-neoliberal social bond might look like, my claim is that the revolt embodied that from the outset. I subsequently define critical subjectivities in line with Simon Critchley's work. This allows me to determine in greater detail the relevance of critical scholars in exploring identification with emancipatory events. Finally, I outline the psychoanalytic approach that I will adopt in the following chapters. I clarify how the Lacanian notions of desire, fantasy, the Other, imaginary, and symbolic enable me to empirically study the libidinal economy of identification with the *estallido*. I also show how my approach closely aligns with other perspectives on emancipatory events, such as Kristin Ross' treatment of the Paris Commune.

The analysis of my empirical material begins with Chapter 3. Here, I offer an interpretation of the psychic labour involved in countering the misrecognition coming from the main motto of the revolt, 'Chile woke up'. I reconstruct the *fantasy of sleeplessness* as an imaginary framework that allows subjects to reclaim a sense of self-recognition in response to the overwhelming call of the revolt. Drawing on a non-pathological theory of hallucinations, I explore the parallels between the command to wake up from the neoliberal slumber and the logic of the unchained signifier to understand the psychic strain involved in identifying with the emancipatory call of the *estallido*. The logic of the unchained signifier underscores a circle that is hard to psychically square: we know that we are awake, but we do not know what we have woken up to. My interpretation suggests that, faced with these difficulties, this fantasy allows the subject to identify with the caller (the Other of the *estallido*) rather than with its call.

Chapter 4 examines the visual oversaturation of the revolt. In an effort to counter media disinformation and document police brutality, video recordings became nearly ubiquitous during the *estallido*. My interpretation shows the unconscious effects of this constant pressure to record everything at all times through the *fantasy of immediacy*. Drawing on the relentless attempt to see 'everything' and the homophony between the words duty (*deber*), indebtedness (*deber*) and to see (*de-ver*), I examine how a distinctive conception of mediation—both as falsehood and as external—is constructed and contrasted with the presumed immediacy of these recordings. In this context, the act of seeing becomes libidinised, enabling subjects to 'find' themselves within the revolt.

Chapter 5 delves into the contradictory ways in which activity and passivity were psychically registered during the revolt, particularly in the context of academic writing. Subjects often engaged in a series of mental gymnastics to allow themselves to write while simultaneously asserting that they did not, as this seemed out of bounds. The *fantasy of impotence* serves as an imaginary narrative that permits the circulation of this desire in a compromised form, granting subjects a sense of self-recognition. This unconscious strategy ultimately creates a symbolic divide between a transgressive other, who enjoys writing, and those who acknowledge the prohibition against writing (but still do it). My interpretation underscores the counterintuitive and ambivalent allure of impotence as a figure of identification.

Chapter 6 explores the imaginary underpinnings of sociology in Chile. Although only two sociologists were included in my sample, 'sociology' as a signifier emerged in nearly every interview. The excessive discursive authority of this signifier in determining what counts as valid knowledge prompted an analysis of its libidinal dimension during the revolt. My interpretation reveals an ambivalent relationship to change, particularly when those advocating for transformation hold a dominant position in the circulation and validation of transformative knowledge. The *fantasy of clairvoyance* highlights how social change can be experienced as a loss and how the lost object can be entirely imaginary. The eroticisation of sociology as a signifier in my empirical material offers insight into the psychic struggle to accept the waning of phallic authority in the face of social change.

Chapter 7 provides an in-depth interpretation of the relationship to power during the *estallido*. One of the most striking aspects of my interviews is that power is almost invariably an attribute of the Other, particularly the perceived machinations of neoliberal academia. This creates a paradox: during one of the most politically empowering events in the country's history, subjects feel compelled to relinquish their power. The challenge is that most of the academics I interviewed hold objective embodiments of power. This power must therefore circulate in ways that render it psychically bearable. The *fantasy of powerlessness* stages a scenario where power is imaginarily constructed as its absence.

Chapter 8 presents the main conclusions of my study. First, I outline the 'dignity' of fantasy for the study of emancipatory identifications. Second, I explore the commonalities among the fantasies I reconstructed, suggesting that my findings point to a continuity rather than a rupture with the libidinal economy of neoliberalism in the *estallido*. Drawing on Todd McGowan's idea of 'pure excess' as the defining feature of capitalism's libidinal economy, I argue that this continuity lies in the excessive unconscious responses to the already excessive call of the Other. Finally, I use these findings to contribute to a conceptual discussion on the possibility of emancipatory fantasies.

References

Almeida, P., & Pérez, A. (2022). *Collective Resistance to Neoliberalism.* Cambridge University Press.

Althusser, L. (2020). *What is to be Done?* Polity.

Asún, R., Rdz-Navarro, K., & Tintaya, M. (2020). ¿Por qué surgen los estallidos sociales? Emociones, redes interpersonales, rituales y participación en protestas. *Última Década, 54*, 5–40.

Atria, F., Larraín, G., Benavente, J. M., Couso, J., & Joignant, A. (2014). *El Otro Modelo: Del Orden Neoliberal al Régimen de lo Público.* Debate.

Ballard, R., & Barnett, C. (Eds.). (2023). *The Routledge Handbook of Social Change*. Routledge.

Barder, A. (2013). American Hegemony Comes Home: The Chilean Laboratory and the Neoliberalization of the United States. *Alternatives: Global, Local, Political, 38*(2), 103–121.

Berardi, F. (2021). *The Third Unconscious*. Verso.

Bevins, V. (2023). *If We Burn: The Mass Protest Decade and the Missing Revolution*. Wildfire.

Bloom, P. (2016). Work as the Contemporary Limit of Life: Capitalism, the Death Drive, and the Lethal Fantasy of 'Work-life Balance.' *Organization, 23*(4), 588–606.

Bottici, C. (2014). *Imaginal Politics: Images Beyond Imagination and the Imaginary*. Columbia University Press.

Bracher, M. (1993). *Lacan, Discourse, and Social Change: A Psychoanalytic Cultural Criticism*. Cornell University Press.

Bröckling, U. (2015). *The Entrepreneurial Self: Fabricating a New Type of Subject*. SAGE Publications.

Browne, C., & Diehl, P. (2019). Conceptualising the Political Imaginary: An Introduction to the Special Issue. *Social Epistemology, 33*(5), 393–397.

Brunner, J. (1998). Malestar en la sociedad chilena: ¿De qué, exactamente, estamos hablando? *Estudios Públicos, 72*, 173–198.

Bucci, F., Romelli, K., & Vanheule, S. (2022). Lacanian Discourse Analysis and Emotional Textual Analysis Compared: New Proposals on Articulating Psychoanalysis and Psychosocial Studies. *Psychoanalysis, Culture & Society, 27*(2–3), 163–180.

Cahill, D. (2014). *The End of Laissez-Faire?* Edward Elgar.

Castiglia, C. (2017a). Hope for Critique? In E. Anker & R. Felski (Eds.), *Critique and Postcritique*. Duke University Press.

Castiglia, C. (2017b). *The Practices of Hope. Literary Criticism in Disenchanted Times*. New York University Press.

Castillo, A. (2019). *Asamblea de los Cuerpos*. London: Sangría Editora.

Copjec, J. (2015). *Read my Desire*. Verso.

Cortés, A. (2022). *Chile, el Fin del Mito. Estallido, Pandemia y Ruptura Constituyente*. RIL Editores.

Daly, G. (1999). Ideology and its Paradoxes: Dimensions of Fantasy and Enjoyment. *Journal of Political Ideologies, 4*(2), 219–238.

Dardot, P. (2023). *La Memoria del Futuro, Chile 2019–2022*. Editorial Gedisa.

Dardot, P., & Laval, C. (2017). *The New Way of the World: On Neoliberal Society*. Verso.

Duncombe, S., & Harrebye, S. (2022). Political Imagination. In V. Glăveanu (Ed.), *The Palgrave Encyclopedia of the Possible*. Palgrave Macmillan.

Edwards, S. (2019, November 30). *Chile's Insurgency and the End of Neoliberalism*. Centre for Economic Policy Research (Online). https://cepr.org/voxeu/columns/chiles-insurgency-and-end-neoliberalism.

Ferretti, P., & Dragnic, M. (2020). Chile: La Revuelta en el Laboratorio Neoliberal. In O. Grau, L. Follegati & S. Aguilera (Coords.), *Escrituras Feministas en la Revuelta*. LOM Ediciones.

Frosh, S., Vyrgioti, M., & Walsh, J. (2024). *The Palgrave Handbook of Psychosocial Studies*. Palgrave Macmillan.

Galende, F. (2020). Pueblo, Arte, Sublevación. In F. Gaspar & G. Jarpa (Eds.), *Los Futuros Imaginados*. Vicerrectoría de Investigación y Desarrollo, Universidad de Chile.

Glynos, J. (2001). The Grip of Ideology: A Lacanian Approach to the Theory of Ideology. *Journal of Political Ideologies, 6*(2), 191–214.

Glynos, J. (2021). Critical Fantasy Studies. *Journal of Language and Politics, 20*(1), 95–111.

Glynos, J., Oliveira, G., & Burity, J. (2019). Critical Fantasy Studies: Neoliberalism, Education and Identification. An Interview with Jason Glynos. *Série-Estudos, 24*(52), 145–170.

Glynos, J., & Stavrakakis, Y. (2008). Lacan and Political Subjectivity: Fantasy and Enjoyment in Psychoanalysis and Political Theory. *Subjectivity, 24*(1), 256–274.

Hoedemaekers, C. (2019). The Fantasy of Control: Behaviourist Transgressions of Neoliberal Subjectivity. *Psychoanalysis, Culture & Society, 24*(3), 303–322.

Hook, D. (2013). Tracking the Lacanian Unconscious in Language. *Psychodynamic Practice, 19*(1), 38–54.

Hook, D. (2020). White Anxiety in (Post)apartheid South Africa. *Psychoanalysis, Culture & Society, 25*(4), 612–631.

Kapoor, I. (2020). *Confronting Desire*. Cornell University Press.

Kapoor, I., Fridell, G., Sioh, M., & de Vries, P. (2023). *Global Libidinal Economy*. SUNY Press.

Karmy, R. (2019). *El Porvenir Se Hereda. Fragmentos de un Chile Sublevado*. Sangría Editora.

Karmy, R. (2020). *Intifada: Una Topología de la Imaginación Popular*. Ediciones Metales Pesados.

Kornbluh, A. (2022). Solidarity Words. *Differences, 33*(2–3), 33–50.

Lacan, J. (2017). *The Seminar of Jacques Lacan, Book V: Formations of the Unconscious*. Polity.

Leader, D. (2021). *Jouissance Sexuality, Suffering and Satisfaction*. Polity.
Landaeta, L., & Herrero, V. (2021). *La Revuelta. Las Semanas de Octubre que Estremecieron Chile*. Planeta.
Lapping, C. (2011). *Psychoanalysis in Social Research*. Routledge.
Loick, D. (2018). If You're a Critical Theorist, How Come You Work for a University? *Critical Horizons, 19*(3), 233–245.
Martuccelli, D. (2019). El largo Octubre Chileno. Bitácora Sociológica. In K. Araujo (Ed.), *Hilos Tensados. Para Leer el Octubre Chileno*. Editorial USACH.
Marx, K. (1978). Economic and Philosophic Manuscripts of 1844. In R. Tucker (Ed.), *The Marx-Engels Reader*. W. W. Norton & Company.
Marx, K., & Engels, F. (1998). *The German Ideology*. Prometheus Books.
McGowan, T. (2022). Mainstreaming Fantasy: Politics Without Reserve. *Differences, 33*(2–3), 177–197.
McGowan, T. (2024). *Embracing Alienation: Why We Shouldn't Try to Find Ourselves*. Repeater Books.
Moyano, C. (2021). Cartografía Genealógica de las 'Narrativas del Malestar': El Chile de la Transición entre 1990–1998. *Revista De Historia, 28*(1), 482–513.
Neill, C. (2013). Breaking the text: An Introduction to Lacanian Discourse Analysis. *Theory & Psychology, 23*(3), 334–350.
Nunes, R. (2021). *Neither Vertical nor Horizontal*. Verso.
Palacios, M. (2011). A psychosocial Interpretation of Political Violence: Chile 1970–1973. *Psychoanalysis, Culture & Society, 16*(3), 244–260.
Patton, M. (2002). *Qualitative Research and Evaluation Methods* (3rd ed.). SAGE Publications.
Phillips, A. (2018). Looking at Obstacles. In *One Way and Another: New and Selected Essays*. Penguin.
Phillips, A. (2021). *On Wanting to Change*. Penguin.
Proctor, H. (2024). *Burnout: The Emotional Experience of Political Defeat*. Verso.
Rancière, J. (2010). *La Noche de los Proletarios: Archivos del Sueño Obrero*. Tinta Limón.
Rodríguez, J. P. (2020). *Resisting Neoliberal Capitalism in Chile: The Possibility of Social Critique*. Palgrave Macmillan.
Ronderos, S., & Glynos, J. (2022). Anti-populist Fantasies: Interrogating Veja's Discursive Constructions, from Lula to Bolsonaro. *Critical Discourse Studies, 20*(6), 618–642.
Ross, K. (2024). *The commune Form: The Transformation of Everyday Life*. Verso.
Ruiz, C. (2020). *Octubre Chileno. La Irrupción de un Nuevo Pueblo*. Taurus.

Ruiz, C., & Boccardo, G. (2015). *Los Chilenos Bajo el Neoliberalismo. Clases y Conflicto Social*. Fundación Nodo XXI/El Desconcierto.
Ruti, M. (2012). Reading Lacan as a Social Critic: What it Means not to cede on one's desire. *Angelaki, 17*(1), 69–81.
Ruti, M. (2018). *Distillations: Theory, Ethics, Affect*. Bloomsbury Academic.
Sánchez, G. (2025). Critique, Postcritique and the Pandemoniac Horizon. *Parallax, 30*(2), 227–244.
Sánchez, G., Valenzuela, F., & Sanfuentes, M. (2024). In pursuit of (post-)bureaucratic Promises: Analyzing the Logics of Career Self-management Discourse at a Privatized Company. *Scandinavian Journal of Management, 40*(1), Article 101318.
Somma, N., Garreton, M., Campos, T., & Joignant, A. (2020). Radiografia del estallido social. In A. Joignant, N. Somma, M. Garretón, & T. Campos (Eds.), *Informe Anual Observatorio de Conflictos*. COES Chile.
Stavrakakis, Y. (2019). Introduction. In Y. Stavrakakis (Ed.), *Routledge Handbook of Psychoanalytic Political Theory*. Routledge.
Thayer, W. (2023). Revolt/performance: The Performative Pause. *The South Atlantic Quarterly, 122*(4), 849–854.
Thielemann, L. (2020). Notas para la historia de un desencuentro en la revuelta. Sobre alianzas sociales, izquierdas y una década de luchas sociales. Chile, 2011–2020. *Revista Némesis, 16*, 109–119.
Vera, A. (Ed.). (2017). *Malestar Social y Desigualdades en Chile*. Ediciones Universidad Alberto Hurtado.
Villalobos-Ruminott, S. (2020). Chilean Revolts and the Crisis of Neoliberal Governance. *Radical Philosophy, 2*(7), 9–16.
Žižek, S. (1997). *The Plague of Fantasies*. Verso.
Zupančič, A. (2000). *Ethics of the Real*. Verso.

2
Answering the Desiring Call of the Revolt

This chapter develops a conceptual and methodological framework for studying identification with emancipatory events. Previously, I introduced readers to the Chilean *estallido* and sought to persuade them that Lacanian psychoanalysis enables us to steer away from restorative approaches and power-centred models. I argued that focusing on the identification of critical scholars with 'the experience of the end of neoliberalism' (Castillo, 2019, p. 42) can empirically demonstrate that such an experience cannot be adequately understood either by assuming a purely negative role of alienation or by prioritising power relations. Taking this further, the first part of this chapter establishes the conceptual grounds upon which this critical subject is defined. Drawing on Simon Critchley (2008), I maintain that the proximity of Chilean critical scholars to neoliberalism as a signifier is precisely what makes them suitable candidates for studying the libidinal economy of the revolt. As Danilo Martuccelli (2021, p. 6) has observed: 'In spite of the diversity of interpretations the *estallido* has given rise to, neoliberalism is always, in one way or another, the overall framework of analysis'. I endeavour to show that this is not merely an epistemological choice but

G. Sánchez, *A Rebel Unconscious*, Studies in the Psychosocial,
https://doi.org/10.1007/978-3-032-12275-9_2

something closer to an existential position: critical subjects are simultaneously constituted and divided by this cherished obstacle. By pushing Chileans to situate themselves 'in relation to a desired place in the future' that is no longer neoliberal (Dardot, 2023, p. 226), the revolt set in motion an ambivalent psychic economy—particularly evident, though not exclusively so, among critical scholars.

That the *estallido* 'pushed' Chileans to identify with a post-neoliberal social bond must be taken literally. The second part of this chapter lays out the notions that underpin the conceptualisation of this push—desire, fantasy, Other, imaginary, and symbolic—together with the methodological principles that render them empirically graspable. From another angle, the *estallido* has also been read as a call or invitation to social change. By way of example, researchers have explored the power of memory to understand how the revolt's 'ethical imperative to be part of a possibility for societal change' took hold (Aedo et al., 2024, p. 200). The claim here is that the political subjectivation of the popular uprising did not operate through conventional means—such as political militancy or ideology—but by activating subterranean memories, particularly those linked to the dictatorship. These memories became a reservoir of meaning Chileans drew upon when experiencing the ethical call of the revolt, shaping the desire for 'total and systematic immersion' in the events (p. 192). My approach departs from this conceptualisation of the revolt's push, contending that the desire for social change is far less straightforward than this image suggests. Just as desire is not the felicitous encounter between a dormant disposition and its activation, so meaning and recognition do not exhaust the experience of identification. The aim of my conceptualisation is to show that misrecognition is not accidental but constitutive of identification itself. This invites us to explore how individuals psychically coped with the fact that, rather than a one-to-one, fully meaningful activation, at times the revolt's call felt senseless.

The chapter closes by fleshing out the structural similarities between my approach and other attempts to study identification with emancipatory events. Kristin Ross' (2016, 2023, 2024) systematic exploration of the Paris Commune of 1871 closely aligns with my interpretation of the *estallido*. She approaches the Commune's archives to trace the movement of the literal words put into circulation by the communards, showing how certain privileged terms exerted an interpellative force upon them. Put differently, she tracks how these words became the vehicle through which the call to identify with social change was launched. The virtue of her analysis lies in her strictly symbolic focus, which eloquently illustrates the subjective implications of the materiality of the signifier for my own study (Lapping, 2016). In order to empirically grasp the unconscious dynamics at play in the identification with the *estallido*, interpretation must take as its object the words deployed to make sense of the experience, rather than their intended meaning. Materiality here refers to words in isolation: sounds, shapes, homophonies, and double entendres are among the elements that come to the fore for Lacanian psychoanalysis. Just as Ross pays close attention to words that may seem purely decorative to draw political lessons from the Commune, I attend to the words in the orbit of the *estallido* to derive unconscious ones.

Who Answers the Emancipatory Call?

The previous chapter underscored the differences between my perspective on the subject and approaches to subjectivity predicated upon power, as represented by critiques of the 'neoliberal subject'. It is time to develop this insight further by providing the foundations of the concept of the subject I work with. While 'subjectivity' and 'subject' tend to be used interchangeably, there are important theoretical and practical discrepancies in deploying each term. What prompts the overlapping of both notions is the assumption that, when it comes to understanding social phenomena, we cannot take the human being as our immediate referent. Neither subjectivity nor the subject, therefore, are merely fancier words for the individual. They call attention to processes that shape our very experience as individuals, which is not a spontaneous occurrence. So far, so good. Now, for researchers aligned with the concept of subjectivity, the point is that 'the modern individual is not just a fact of our humanity but is rather a historical product of disciplinary power in its overall form as well as in the specifics of the subject-positions we have inherited' (Heyes, 2011, p. 171). Here is where the discrepancies bubble up.

The emphasis of power-centred models on history, discipline, and positionality implies that society can be understood as a realm of competing forces trying to establish where individuals should be and how they should behave. We are the historical product of those forces, either because we embrace a particular subjectivity or because we refuse its command. Therefore, studying subjectivity becomes a matter of tracing the technologies that makes us be in a certain way and obstruct our path to be otherwise. When we incorporate the idea that emancipatory events such as the *estallido* can be experienced as a push or a call, the emphasis on positionality carries the assumption that this can only have a positive result—the call always reaches its target. In this respect, what appears to be so poignant about the subjectivation of the revolt for Aedo et al. (2024) is that individuals without a track record of political militancy were able to adopt a radical position with which they identified fully. They broke free from the neoliberal disciplinary power and its depoliticising effects to become the embodiment of an alternative, resisting subjectivity. Inasmuch as the analysis brings to the fore the role of historical forces, the *estallido* is thus understood as an event that made us shift from a retrograde position to a resisting one.

When we approach this emancipatory call from the perspective of the subject tied to the psychoanalytic tradition, we arrive at a very different conclusion. For Joan Copjec (2015), the reduction of society to its internal networks of power and knowledge is a historicist pitfall that obfuscates the productive role of negativity in our identifications. This difference can be better understood by examining the processes through which desire is brought into being and rendered intelligible within the social field. As per power-centred theorists, ours is not a society that forbids desire but rather instigates it, and the problem is that we cannot rid ourselves of the insidiousness of this mandate. For Copjec, this means that desire is a twofold realisation or positivity. On the one hand, desire is an actual state allowed by society. On the other, since we cannot but have desires, only external forces can prevent their fulfilment. Either way, 'the destiny of desire is realization, unless it is prohibited by something outside it' (Copjec, 2015, p. 24). Conceptually, desire for psychoanalysis has a completely different origin. Desire is correlative to the emergence of the subject precisely because it is something that has effects despite being unrealised—the subject is not an individual *with* a historically determined kind of desire, but an entity that is *at odds with* its own desire regardless of its historical modulation. This is the case since the subject

> [...] does not come into being as the realization of a possibility opened up by the law of the Other. It is rather an impossibility that is crucial to the constitution of the subject – the impossibility, precisely, of any ultimate confirmation from the Other. The subject emerges, as a result, as a desiring being, that is to say, an effect of the law but certainly not a realization of it, since desire as such can never be conceived as a realization. Desire fills no possibility but seeks after an impossibility; this makes desire always, constitutionally, contentless. (Copjec, 2015, p. 36)

Disentangling effect from realisation allows us to account for negativity in the study of desire and identification. The Other—which can be temporarily defined as the set of implicit rules organising society—can never grant secure places for individuals to occupy, not even within overtly oppressive regimes. Where subjectivity finds either capture *or* resistance, the subject encounters both doubt *and* anxiety. Unlike subjectivity, the subject is not conditional on meaning but upon meaninglessness; at its core, we find an ineradicable experience of misrecognition due to the fact that the Other is an insubstantial entity that cannot uphold our being. From this angle, desire and identification are not things that we have or resist, which would turn them into resources we can consciously leverage. For Lacanian psychoanalysis, desire 'is the problem rather than the solution' (McGowan, 2016, p. 48). As I will develop later, the psychoanalytic procedure is not to solve problems but to learn to see how the very form of the problem contains its solution. The challenge ahead lies in articulating a conceptualisation of the subject that is not defined through its opposition to subjectivity, but rather affirms its singularity in terms of constitutive misrecognition and its relation to lack.

Since the wager of my study is that the misrecognition of the *estallido*'s emancipatory call is particularly evident among critical scholars,

Simon Critchley's ethico-political notion of the subject is a good place to start. His point of departure is that the fundamental political experience is disappointment. This is the case because the realisation that we live in a violently unjust world is the first political discernment; it is what prompts engagements with different conceptions of justice. For his theoretical project, the goal is to find a notion of ethics that can operate as a motivational force to face contemporary forms of disappointment. In this sense, Critchley (2008, p. 10) provides the following definition: 'A subject is the name for the way in which a self binds itself to some conception of the good and shapes its subjectivity in relation to that good'. Two aspects of this definition demand clarification. First, this is not a mechanism to manufacture moral selves, but a way of pointing out that there is an ethical kernel in the subject, expressed in the embracement of a good. Second, the nature of such good is certainly not predefined, meaning that it varies from subject to subject. However, it invariably has a paradoxical effect. If the condition of possibility for a subject is this self-binding to a good, the latter is expressed through an incommensurate demand that overflows the subject. This means that the ethical demand the subject attaches itself to is both its condition of possibility and impossibility.

Based on the above, the subject is not a pre-given existence—it is not simply an individual—but something one becomes by attaching oneself to an impossible, hyperbolic demand for justice. This is thus an internally divided subject; something that is in excess of itself. Consequently, even if a decision is at the heart of subject formation, self-transparency can never be attained. This is due to the circularity of ethical experience: 'The point is that the demand is not somehow objectively given in the state of affairs. Rather, the demand is only felt *as* a demand for the self who approves of it' (Critchley, 2008, p. 18). We can perceive how Critchley conceptualises a notion of the subject aligned with the radical contingency of the *estallido*: in the same way that the revolt is an anti-neoliberal event that cannot be sufficiently explained by neoliberalism, subject formation cannot be sufficiently explained by the approval of a particular demand since these moments are one and the same thing; demand and approval emerge in unison. The demand for the good that stands as the principle of the subject's articulation is deducible from, but not reducible to, the situation. When a subject feels 'pushed' in a certain way, i.e., to act in conformity with a good, it means that fidelity to a sort of forced choice is at play. The demand is experienced as the only way forward and this creates an opacity within the subject.

There are multiple advantages to working with the notion of the subject advanced by Critchley. First, as mentioned, this ethical definition of the subject is fully compatible with the contingency of the *estallido*. To use a more technical term, the moment of undecidability at stake in the revolt is also operative in the subject. Second, it enables me to problematise the alleged self-recognition of critical scholars in their practice. Inasmuch as the demand around which the subject is articulated is excessive, transparent agency becomes an unachievable outcome. As a result, desire and identification cannot be understood as the straightforward fulfilment of social mandates. Third, Critchley's notion rests on the possibility of counteracting political disappointment, which is precisely what defines the *estallido*. A popular uprising appears as one of the most salient demands for political justice. Crucially, the fact that the demand emerging from such a context is irreducible to the situation not only implies that it is ultimately unfulfillable, but also that it constitutes 'a situated demand that is addressed, in principle, to everyone and hence universal' (Critchley, 2008, p. 42). To continue with the language I have been using: feeling the revolt's call is not optional, what is optional is the response.

Through a brief historical detour, we will be in a position to put this definition of the subject to use in the context of the *estallido*. The humanities and social sciences in Latin America have historically been endowed with a utopic horizon of social change, organised around what Manuel Antonio Garretón (2015) calls 'limit concepts'—that is, a desired destination towards which society must advance. The social sciences began to consolidate in the region during the 1960s, a period defined by a clear diagnosis of social transformation: Latin America was either an underdeveloped or a dependent capitalist society. Consequently, academic labour was expected to inform the stages required to achieve development or the conditions to stage a revolution. The limit concepts of 'development' and 'socialism' were the competing goods orienting the self-shaping of academics during this period. For the inchoate field of the social sciences, the challenge was therefore not so much theoretical as professional. The clarity regarding the desired horizon nonetheless lacked a professionalised community of researchers as its counterpart, bearing in mind that the social sciences were still in the making. According to Garretón (2015, p. 160), who was part of this process, 'it was clear what world we were facing and how we wanted to change it, but we did not know what we were as social scientists'.

For the generations of scholars populating the Chilean universities after the dictatorship (1973–1990), anti-neoliberalism slowly yet steadily replaced development and socialism as the limit concepts orienting the academic experience. To return to Critchley, neoliberalism became the notion that underpinned the realisation that we live in a violently unjust world. The privileged position that neoliberalism came to occupy within academia allowed it to almost single-handedly organise critical identifications. As Garretón (2015, p. 161) succinctly puts it, neoliberalism became 'the single dominant principle of totality in society, [...] the sole explanation of all evils'. Even studies that seek to challenge the overbearing explanatory authority of neoliberalism end up reaffirming its status as the limit concept of contemporary Chilean academia. According to Ismael Puga (2020), rather than producing a profound cultural transformation reflected in entrepreneurial mindsets and lifestyles, neoliberalism has led instead to rational or practical adaptations to material conditions. In his view, the very belief among scholars that neoliberalism has radically reshaped Chilean subjectivity ends up lending it an appearance of solidity. Considering this, Puga (2020, p. 229) concludes that 'Chileans, like social scientists, perceive a fantasy neoliberal consensus'.

This cursory historical overview suffices to illustrate the role that neoliberalism has played in shaping critical identities within Chilean academia. As a consequence, the critical scholars who experienced the *estallido* can be defined as *a way of self-binding to a post-neoliberal society and the ensuing attempts to shape themselves in relation to this good*. It should now be clear why I chose to focus on their experiences to explore the role of alienation in emancipatory identifications. When we make room for the idea that desire is not the positive realisation of a historical position, the post-neoliberal experience brought about by the *estallido* cannot be straightforwardly interpreted as the fulfilment of a desire. And, despite appearances, this is most evident among those whose identities are bound up with labouring towards a post-neoliberal society. At this precise point, however, Critchley's theory requires supplementation. While he is right to argue that the excessiveness of the good renders it impossible for the subject to find self-realisation in the binding process, he does not explicitly link this excess to lack or structural alienation. Once we make this connection, we realise that we cannot find ourselves in the good because its excessiveness functions as an imaginary placeholder—one that makes bearable the alienation or misrecognition we receive from the Other. In line with Copjec, we cling to the good because there is no ultimate confirmation from the Other that we are what we are. In embracing the good, we elevate a signifier to a different status in order to cope with this absence of confirmation.

So, who answered the emancipatory call of the *estallido*? Not a positive subjectivity who finally found its long-yearned-for place in the world, but a subject who has lost the imaginary good that had hitherto organised its self-shaping. In short, an alienated entity that must grapple with its lack of self-identity—a *way* of self-binding without anything to bind itself to. We can now see why the formulation of the cherished obstacle that I borrow from Phillips (2018) is so apt: the fact that neoliberalism can be an obstacle to social justice does not preclude it from simultaneously being a cherished good organising our psychic economy. Once we treat neoliberalism as a signifier, we are in a position to explore this economy. And since critical scholars depend so heavily on this cherished obstacle, studying their experience of alienation amid the *estallido* stands as an opportunity to examine the unconscious dynamics of emancipatory identification. From this angle, staging a post-neoliberal experience can be understood as a traumatic event, as it exposes the distance we bear to ourselves; the confirmation that there is no confirmation from the Other.

If the above seems counterintuitive, it is only because we have come to believe that alienation and oppression are one and the same. No one has done more in recent years to debunk this fraudulent correlation than Todd McGowan (2024). To do so, he theorises alienation as foundational, meaning that it is not contingent upon an original, non-alienated situation. Insofar as we relate to ourselves and to the world through language, which is external to us, it is distance and not immediacy that sustains our existence. The case is not that we originally possessed something and historical forces separated us from it—the only original thing we ever had was this separation from ourselves, as the frail verification of who we are invariably comes from outside. This is the reason why identification exists in the first place: 'Although the signifier forms the basis for symbolic identity, it also highlights a crack within the natural being that forces the subject to take up a position relative to what it is' (McGowan, 2024, p. 14).

Despite appearances, this original lack of self-identity is emancipatory. If we do not fully coincide with the historical conditions within which we come to be—if there is more than just successful acquiescence or successful resistance—then we can never be wholly determined by them. As McGowan (2024, p. 3) summarises it: 'I am never identical with the position into which I am born. This gives me the possibility of relating to this position critically'. Is this not precisely what the experience of the end of neoliberalism elicited by the *estallido* was all about? The revolt exposed our lack of self-identity, forcing us to take up a position relative to what we are. This is the alienating yet emancipatory call of the *estallido*—a universal call. Due to their investment in neoliberalism as a signifier, the responses of critical scholars become a privileged locus for studying the libidinal reorganisation of our self-distancing, as well as the ways in which confirmation from the Other is sought in emancipatory settings.

The Revolt's Desire

For the sake of simplicity, I referred earlier to the Other as the set of implicit rules organising society. This characterisation might be readily accepted by Lacanian scholars, yet I believe it only approximates what Lacan sought to conceptualise. Moreover, the fact that such a definition is customarily taken as precise renders the concept of the Other a source of severe epistemological and political misunderstanding. Let me offer two examples. For Lee Edelman (2004), politics is a realm of imaginary relations competing for the fulfilment of symbolic identifications. Here, the alienating aspect of the signifier is concealed while history follows the rhythm of desire rather than the drive, the source of radical negativity. Thus, instead of inhabiting the space of the Other, Edelman urges us to divest ourselves of identity by embracing the drive, 'the negativity opposed to every form of social viability' (p. 9). Jodi Dean's otherwise incisive analysis of neofeudalism presents a wholly different kind of confusion. Among the features defining neofeudalism, she identifies the parcellation of sovereignty into small, privatised pockets. She contends that the fragmentation of the symbolic order is correlative to this parcellation of sovereignty, resulting in a concomitant parcellation of the Other. Ultimately, she sees this reflected in the contemporary sentiment that 'nobody cares', which for her marks the decline of symbolic efficiency: 'There's no big Other who cares or who sees us caring' (Dean, 2025, p. 107).

When the Other is equated with society or sociality, we risk falling prey to the idea that it can simply be replaced with something else (like Edelman proposes), or that its foundations have been eroded to such an extent that it has effectively disappeared (like Dean suggests). Such positions close the door to another possibility: the Other as an emancipatory place, which is my claim. The idea that the Other can be bypassed or worn so thin as to become non-existent is, I contend, theoretically unfounded. The reason is that, if either alternative were viable, psychoanalysis would be deprived of all interpretive value whatsoever. Lacan is remarkably consistent on this point. As early as *Seminar I* (1991, p. 171), he asserts that 'the subject inhabits the world of the symbol [...]. That is why his desire is susceptible to the mediation of recognition'. In *Seminar III* (1997a, p. 168), Lacan describes the Other as the place 'where the subject recognizes himself and gets himself recognized'. In *Seminar IV* (2020, p. 100), he insists that what is essential in the unconscious is 'the subject's relation to the Other as such'. In *Seminar VI* (2019, p. 15) he is even more explicit: 'The subject asks the Other what he wants. The question is asked from the place where the subject first encounters desire, desire being initially the Other's desire'. And in *Seminar VII* (1997b, p. 309), we find the well-known formulation that 'desire of man is the desire of the Other', which is repeated in the same terms, among other places, in *Seminar XI* (1998, p. 38) and in *Seminar XVII* (2007, p. 61). Therefore, unless we are willing to do away with both the unconscious and desire, the Other is not a matter of preference but the fulcrum of psychoanalytic interpretation.

At a terminological level, we face the obvious fact that, had Lacan intended the Other to be synonymous with the social or sociality, he would not have found it necessary to coin a specific concept. More fundamentally though, the singularity of the Other can be discerned in the way Lacan employs the term 'recognition'. The following is a key excerpt from *Seminar III*:

> In true speech the Other is that before which you make yourself recognized. But you can make yourself recognized by it only because it is recognized first. It has to be recognized for you to be able to make yourself recognized [...]. It is through recognizing it that you institute it [the Other], and not as a pure and simple element of reality, a pawn, a puppet, but as an irreducible absolute, on whose existence as subject the very value of the speech in which you get yourself recognized depends. Something gets born there. (Lacan, 1997a, p. 51)

The Other is not merely an element of reality in which we can recognise ourselves because, for psychoanalysis, *what we must first recognise is recognition as such*. This crucial step is elided in sociological accounts of identification and therein lies the reason why the Other allows us to explore a properly psychoanalytic dynamic. The Other is not directly the social or sociality, but the psychic inscription of the necessity of attaining recognition from an external entity. Put concisely, the Other is instituted when the recognition of recognition has occurred. This process has an unconscious upshot, and it is neither oppressive nor optional; it is simply a structural feature of our symbolic existence.

Granting the *estallido* the status of the Other allows us to study the recognition of recognition in emancipatory events. When I emphasise the experience of the end of neoliberalism, or draw on Rancière's idea of living neoliberalism according to the logic of post-neoliberalism, I am certainly not suggesting that neoliberalism was effaced from Chile. My point, rather, is that the revolt can be regarded as emancipatory only insofar as it transformed the way in which we had hitherto internalised the recognition of recognition. Emancipation, from a psychoanalytic point of view, should be studied in terms of the responses we, as alienated subjects, produce in order to regain recognition from a new Other. We do not need to inhabit a fully fledged socialist society for emancipatory identifications to take place—what counts as emancipatory is the reencounter with our alienation and the way in which this is reorganised within a new symbolic milieu. Consequently, it is not that the *estallido* brought entrepreneurial mindsets to a halt or suddenly made privatisation and competition obsolete; the point, rather, is that it set in motion a symbolic life with 'phrases that neoliberalism cannot understand, but which are full of meaning for the revolt' (Castillo, 2019, p. 41). A recognition of recognition is a prerequisite for this to occur.

We must now flesh out the consequences of the above. The Other of the revolt is the site from which a new kind of speech derives its value, yet this does not imply that the vicissitudes of recognition have suddenly been overcome. For structural reasons, the call of the *estallido* is one in which we cannot fully confirm ourselves. These structural reasons become apparent in the strange reciprocity at the heart of recognition. We have established that, on account of symbolic mediation, there is a lack of self-identity in the subject—this lack being the origin of unconscious desire. But if this holds, then the Other is not identical with itself either. We must resist the temptation to imagine the Other as a kind of trickster who delights in confusing us for its own amusement. In a way, the Other is unable to confirm who we are because it is itself a lacking entity: 'the Other seems to be split between the site of truth and the site of the desire of the Other. It's the same with the subject' (Lacan, 2008, p. 43). The call of the Other is not authoritative—in the sense of delivering a clear, unambiguous directive to its addressee—but rather *a desiring call*. The distance the subject experiences with itself is also operative in the Other.

The call of the *estallido* reaches us, and by the time we answer it, there is nobody on the Other side of the line. This is why 'we are always asking the Other what he desires' (Lacan, 2008, p. 38). In this post-neoliberal symbolic universe—where things no longer make sense to neoliberalism but are full of meaning for the revolt—we cannot but seek recognition from an incomplete Other, whose response is pierced by gaps and inconsistencies. Recognition, in this sense, becomes a moment of doubt and anxiety rather than one of plenitude or sameness. This is a structurally flawed dynamic, and so 'there is always a residue, a leftover, a stain of traumatic irrationality and senselessness sticking to it' (Žižek, 2008, p. 43). How is it possible, then, that this symbolic inconsistency is experienced as meaningful? Fantasies are responsible for this.

For psychoanalysis, fantasies are narratives or frameworks that render desire readable; they intervene to make misrecognition, as it were, digestible. Fantasies can achieve this because they operate in a different register of our experience: while the Other is embedded in the symbolic dimension of human life, fantasies pertain to the imaginary. In this dimension, 'we always have more and less, a threshold, a margin, continuity. In the symbolic order every element has value through being opposed to another' (Lacan, 1997a, p. 9). The difference between the symbolic and the imaginary is thus correlative to the difference between the signifier and the signified. Without the imaginary, we could never attain even a minimal sense of coherence or continuity, bearing in mind that, in the symbolic, the signifier's only relationship is with another signifier. Simply put, when we turn a signifier into a sign—when we feel that *we are who we are*—there is an imaginary supplement habilitating this experience. Our symbolic world is therefore not directly meaningful but becomes so through the production of imaginary narratives (Glynos, 2021; Žižek, 1997). These are libidinally charged narratives aiming to fill the gaps of recognition by keeping the desire of the Other at bay.

For Lacan (2019, p. 4), 'libido, a notion that lies at the heart of psychoanalytic theory, is nothing but the psychical energy of desire'. Consequently, for our world to be meaningful, the enigma of the desire of the Other is 'solved' by unconsciously energising parts of our symbolic milieu with which we develop a kind of intimate connection. We can understand fantasies as imaginary scenarios whose main purpose is to square a fundamental symbolic antagonism with the subject's conscious life. To produce this effect, fantasies rearrange the terms of a destabilising situation in order to make it psychically bearable for the subject. However, it is crucial not to assume that fantasies are the place where the subject finds self-realisation or where its desire is finally fulfilled. They provide the *location* of desire yet not its realisation, and this is how the subject can cope with its distressing relationship with the desiring call of the Other. When it comes to fantasies, then, what matters most is the obstacle we construct to express our inability to do what we want or to be who we want to be. We libidinise signifiers to erect those obstacles that bring us unconscious satisfaction. In this sense, psychoanalysis is at odds with common sense: 'the desire does not reveal the obstacle, the obstacle reveals the desire' (Phillips, 2018, p. 32).

Why is this so important? Because the self-shaping of critical scholars can give us access to the fantasies that organise the responses to the revolt's desire. Such a study of the libidinal economy of the *estallido* is key to understanding how emancipatory identifications occur. As Anna Kornbluh (2014, p. 137) insightfully notes, 'libidinal' is a term 'for substantifying the workings of desire, [...] designating the foundational structure of psychosocial life'. However, according to her, we remain faithful to the psychoanalytic project only if we take 'economy' as figurative language. This means we must refrain from assuming that there is a single economy regulating our unconscious life. Rather than constituting an immanent order of the psyche, the latter works *like* an economy. Kornbluh's near-forensic approach demonstrates that Freud rarely referred to 'economy' in his writings—an effect largely produced by his translators. He was instead drawn to domestic tropes, evoking the idea that our psyche resembles 'an everyday, everywhere, ongoing process of organizing, putting something to use in a certain way' (2014, p. 144). The term 'economy' is therefore a makeshift at best; a notion that illuminates something which cannot be expressed directly. Our psyche is akin to a resourceful household and the question is how its material is organised, knowing that this is a necessity but there is no necessary organisation.

In this section, I have defined and demonstrated the interrelations between the concepts informing my exploration of the libidinal economy of the *estallido*: the Other, fantasy, unconscious desire, the imaginary, and the symbolic. Anyone minimally familiar with Lacanian theory will have noticed the absence of the real, the third register alongside the symbolic and the imaginary. I have avoided it not because it lacks importance. As I mentioned in the previous chapter, it has become something of a habit among Lacanian scholars to assume that by accounting for rupture, dislocation, interruption, and impossibility—all aspects associated with the real—they can call it a day. This was obviously part of the revolt, and it would be foolish to claim otherwise. The *estallido* evidently dislocated the lives of Chileans, yet applying a conceptual gloss to what is already self-evident adds little, if any, interpretive value to the phenomenon under scrutiny. Moreover, an encounter with the real is not sustainable since it is, properly speaking, a traumatic experience in which the symbolic and the imaginary wane. Some authors outside psychoanalysis claim that this was indeed the experience of the revolt. My study of the libidinal economy of the *estallido* engages with the psychic organisation that emerges in the aftermath of this real dislocation in the form of fantasies—a move that can never root out the disruptiveness of the real. In my view, this is the only way to contribute to the understanding of emancipatory identification without falling prey to the dubious idea that social change is invariably equivalent to rupture.

An Emancipation Already Materially Underway

In this final section, I elaborate on my methodological approach to emancipatory identification. I do so by showing that other researchers have adopted a similar perspective when studying this topic, even if they do not focus on its unconscious dynamics. Kristin Ross is arguably the leading scholar on the Paris Commune of 1871, which has become a sort of benchmark for examining contemporary revolts (Ross, 2024; see also Bernes, 2025). Her primary interest lies in understanding this event both as a concept and as a lived experience. This enterprise leads her to pay close attention to the words the communards used to apprehend their experience of political self-organisation, treating them as her basic analytic unit. Employing a different language, her study brings to the fore the interrelation between the symbolic and the imaginary in studying emancipatory interpellation in a way that aligns with my own approach. By making these parallels explicit, I seek to explain the importance of the idea of the materiality of the signifier, while also illustrating how it informs my approach to the interviews and observations.

For Ross, understanding the everyday life of the Commune requires attention not only to the practice and aims of self-organisation, but also to how self-organisation was named. Reflecting on her approach to the communards' records, she writes: 'I looked closely not only at what they did but at what they thought and said about what they were doing, the words they used, fought over, imported from the past of from distant regions, the words they discarded' (Ross, 2023, p. 257). The Parisian insurgents sought to establish an internationalist organisation capable of producing political identifications beyond the perimeter of the nation-state. To accomplish this, they resorted to a whole array of terms that—just as with the *estallido*—only made sense within a new symbolic milieu. The very notion of 'commune' was one of them: a term that defies 'any precise semantic content, a powerful mix of pre-capitalist and pre- or extra-national desires, equal part of social revolution, local autonomy, and the memory of the insurrectional Commune that had made Paris the capital of revolution in 1792' (Ross, 2016, p. 29). We can perceive how Ross links the desire for social change with the symbolic dimension of its organisation, a process that is always in excess with itself.

Resorting to a slightly different grammar, Ross treats the Commune as the Other, the site from which an emancipatory call was launched. Consequently, the language used by the insurgents to make sense of the uprising conveyed something more than just meaning, 'because the words are an interpellation, a direct second-person address, they create that gap or division in a now, in the contemporary moment constituted by the speech act' (Ross, 2016, p. 16). Since the language of the Commune was calling upon the French people to recognise themselves in an entirely new way, it generated a new temporality in the present. This is the gap or division Ross refers to. However, the conceptualisation I have developed in this chapter allows for another interpretation. The way in which the Commune addressed the French people also confronted them with the psychic challenges of symbolic identification, creating a gap that they had to manoeuvre fantasmatically. This interpretation is supported by the way Ross analyses some of the key words the Commune put into circulation. Among them, '*citoyen*' had a particularly strong grip:

> The name "citoyen," [...] may well be old and originate in another moment of the political past, but its iteration in this instance creates the now of a shared political subjectivization [...] it interpellates listeners to be part of that present. *Citoyen, citoyenne* summons, then, a subject predicated on any number of disidentifications–from the state, the Empire, the police, and the world of the so-called "honnêtes gens." The words are not addressed to the French national citizen. They conjure up an ideal of *la femme libre, l'homme libre*, a non-nationally circumscribed being, and are addressed to and responded to by such listeners accordingly. (Ross, 2016, p. 17)

The Commune, like the *estallido*, was from the outset an emancipatory organisation of the experience, not merely its promise.[1] The communards were thus addressed by the Other of the Commune and, to put it in McGowan's terms, this call compelled them to take up a position in relation to what they are. Using a different conceptual vocabulary, Ross clearly emphasises the interrelation between the imaginary and symbolic registers in order to grasp the desire for social change. Even if she does not explicitly delve into the libidinal economy underpinning the Commune, she is nonetheless attuned to what she calls the 'affective charge' carried by the figures and phrases mobilised by the Parisian insurrection. It is important to note that the words and expressions Ross brings to the fore are not those surrounded by loud fanfare but rather those that appear almost purely ornamental. Another example is the seemingly decorative notion of 'communal luxury'—an expression that appeared in a manifesto drafted by the Artists' Federation under the Commune—from which Ross (2016, 2023) derives a wholesale reconfiguration of the communards' relationship to art and labour. This dimension of emancipatory identification can only be perceived when form takes precedence over content in the work of interpretation.

As I mentioned, Ross' project is not related to psychoanalysis in any explicit way, yet it is clear that her study of emancipatory identification bears a close resemblance to the approach I have advocated in this

[1] This correlates with Maxwell Woods' (2022, p. 167) view of the Chilean revolt: 'In contrast to many readings that see the social explosion as an eruption of discontent that subsequently had to be organized into a blueprint for social relations [...], the social explosion was already offering nascent novel cultural formations'.

chapter. The decisive point is the following: 'The Commune was both rallying cry and the thing itself' (Ross, 2016, p. 20). Jasper Bernes (2025, p. 23) interprets this very line by suggesting that the Commune 'was both a process and an event, both potentiality and actuality'. Based on Ross' symbolic approach, however, I believe we can draw a different conclusion. In my view, Ross is pointing to the divided nature of the Other of the Commune—the fact that, as Lacan puts it, the Other is always split between the site of truth and the site of its desire. The Commune was indeed the everyday life of the communards, what they were meaningfully *doing* in terms of organising an internationalist political bond. But at the same time, it was the symbolic environment in which that doing took place, *and these instances do not coincide with each Other*. The Commune, like the *estallido*, was internally divided, and its call cannot be straightforwardly answered—at least not without a fantasmatic supplement. Therein lies the importance of those mundane words that allowed the communards to navigate the internal split of the Other of the Commune.

The unconscious dimension of emancipatory identification is hinted at in Ross' take on the Commune. All the elements are in place, but their consequences are not developed. To do so, it is necessary to approach the symbolic nature of emancipatory events in a particular fashion. Copjec (2015, p. 8) reminds us that: 'The existence of a thing materially depends on its being articulated in language, for only in this case can it be said to have an objective—that is to say, a verifiable—existence'. Such a formulation already challenges positivist understandings of the material as synonymous with external or tangible reality. But, as we have seen, this creates significant psychic problems for the subject, whose existence is never immediately verifiable through language. For this reason, psychoanalysis does not approach the symbolic as a reservoir of meaning, but intervenes precisely where meaning falters, attending to the meaningless remainder it leaves behind. As Žižek (2000, p. 118) insists, when it comes to psychic life, materiality can never amount to a mere reduction of our inner experience to processes occurring 'out there'; the point is also 'to isolate a "material" traumatic kernel/remainder at the very heart of "psychic life" itself'. Psychoanalytic interpretation identifies the precious words upon which the subject's speech rests and, instead of accepting the value they hold within this speech, separates them in order to approach them *materially*—as signifiers that do not belong to the subject and hence do not always follow its conscious command.

My empirical corpus, composed of interviews and additional observations with Chilean critical scholars, was expressly produced to allow me to intervene at the level of the signifier. The psychoanalytic principle of free association enabled this. Freud (2001, p. 106) described this procedure as follows: 'If I ask someone to tell me what occurs to him in response to a particular element of a dream, I am asking him to surrender himself to free association while keeping an idea in mind as a starting-point'. I am certainly not the first to adapt this principle to social research. Jason Glynos, for instance, has suggested that the aim here is to produce material that has a 'floating character', that is to say, where attempts to impose order on the linguistic exchange, whether by the researcher or the interviewee, give way to a loose and even contradictory concatenation of symbolic chains (Glynos, 2021). The relative undirectedness of the exchange seeks to create an environment in which the participant's ego might be caught 'off guard', stumbling over its own efforts at meaning production. While a state of pure free association is ultimately unattainable (Lapping & Glynos, 2018), the goal is to minimise the directionality in the linguistic exchange and focus interventions on the use of signifiers as they emerge.

Echoing the above, I adapted the principle of free association to ensure that the participants in my study would associate as naturally as possible. Consequently, there was no interview script guiding the exchange; instead, I began each conversation with a single prompt: *Could you please tell me what comes to your mind when I say 'estallido'?* My only aim was for my interviewees to keep associating—letting themselves go wherever the word took them, no matter how rambling or extravagant their thoughts might be. This procedure comes with a range of challenges that cannot be exhaustively addressed here. Perhaps the most difficult one to navigate was that no two interviews were alike. This exercise served as a beautiful reminder of just how easily we 'deviate' from what we are trying to say, and how seemingly random our associations can be. Had someone entered the room five or ten minutes into an interview, it would have been very hard to tell that we were talking about the revolt at all. Chapter 7 offers a good illustration of this. Somehow, talking about cookies and pins can express the ambivalent relationship to power during the *estallido* more effectively than the terms we might conventionally expect in that context.

My interpretation is thus not concerned with the lofty meanings of the revolt's political activation identified by Aedo et al. (2024). Instead, I sought to reconstruct the fantasmatic background within which the self-shaping of these critical subjects took place, by isolating some of the seemingly most *insignificant* elements of their speech. This should be taken as both the most trivial words and those that are devoid of signification, whose sole function is to hold meaning together. The more these subjects got carried away describing something they ostensibly know better than anyone else (their own experience of the *estallido*), the more certain words began to act as grumes or clots in the flow of their speech. As they attempted to offer a coherent narrative, they summoned the Other of the *estallido* as their symbolic guarantor, yet its insubstantial nature prompted the emergence of parallel symbolic associations that show the location of their unconscious desire (Kaufman, 2020). This is the rebelliousness of the unconscious: while they strove to demonstrate how well they fit into the symbolic world inaugurated by the *estallido*, they tripped over the materiality of some of their own words. The more they tried to show that they are who they are because those words are theirs, the more the words themselves rebelled, undermining the very meaning they were meant to uphold.

Let me provide two examples of how I grasped the rebelliousness of the unconscious in my interpretation.[2] In Chapter 4, I dwell on Daniela's experience of the visual manifestation of the *estallido*. This is an aspect that many researchers have picked up on, particularly as it resonated with other revolts around the world. While telling me about the incessant recording of what was happening on the streets, Daniela insisted on the idea that doing this was a 'duty' [*deber*]. At the level of meaning, this seems merely to corroborate the necessity of keeping records of police brutality in order to act upon them legally in the

[2] All participant names used in this book are pseudonyms. To protect privacy, some dates, roles, and locations have been generalised or altered without affecting the substance of the analysis.

future. Yet the manner in which this word emerged suggests something else. Not only can *deber* simultaneously mean 'duty' or 'indebtedness'—which already muddies the waters significantly—but, in the context of widespread visual recording, *deber* sounds exactly like *de-ver*, literally 'to see'. I elaborate on the unconscious effects of this homophony later on. It suffices to note here that the very word which allows Daniela to find her place amid the call of the *estallido* ends up rebelling against this intention *through its materiality as a signifier*. This is precisely what Claudia Lapping (2016, p. 720) invites us to do: to attend to a word's 'sound, the way it is voiced or enacted, and its relation to other signifiers'. Ultimately, it is this kind of attention that enables us to grasp unconscious desire.

In Chapter 5, I explore the strange juxtaposition of activity and passivity amid the *estallido*. A recurrent topic of conversation was the perception that, in spite of all the activity my interviewees engaged in, they nonetheless 'did nothing'. Assessed against their own speech, this was patently incongruous. Furthermore, they sometimes even regarded as impossible something they had nonetheless accomplished (such as writing). Rather than treating this as a contradiction or an attempt to mislead me about the actual state of affairs, I simply took it literally—I probed what those signifiers might be telling me beyond the intended meaning. Accordingly, I interpreted 'doing nothing' not as the absence of activity (its conscious meaning), but as a way of doing something symbolically. I treated 'nothing' as a positive entity in the symbolic register and, consequently, as something that subjects can act upon. This kind of 'doing nothing' opens up an entirely new libidinal dimension in relation to the Other of the *estallido*—a dimension we would overlook were we to remain anchored at the level of meaning. The same applies to my interpretation of 'impotence' in the same fantasmatic space. Once we resist the temptation to take this term as it is intended (as a mere description of how things are), we can see that impotence is less a factual and undesirable condition to be subjected to than an imaginary means to construct an antagonistic divide that makes the revolt's call bearable. This approach allows a reading that goes against common sense, namely, that we can unconsciously enjoy impotence.

The people I interviewed and observed wanted the revolt; they sought to rebel against neoliberalism. Yet when the *estallido* brought the experience of the end of neoliberalism, they received not a confirmation of their identity but the desiring call of the Other of the revolt. The fantasies I reconstruct in the following chapters should be understood as their unconscious negotiations with this call, their psychic struggle with structural misrecognition. *What does the revolt want from me?* This is the enigma of the *estallido* they tried to navigate. Such a phenomenon is not easy to explore in social research, as it runs against the grain of the main presupposition informing qualitative designs. Most handbooks devoted to this matter rehearse different formulations of the same basic postulate: qualitative research is informed by a naturalistic approach, which means that its aim is to arrive at an understanding of the everyday practices of individuals or groups, in their own environment and through their own ways of accounting for them. From this outlook, qualitative research stands as a situated activity of knowledge production premised on the idea that language can grant us access to the meaning-making sustaining individual and collective phenomena (Denzin & Lincoln, 2005; Leavy, 2014; Schwandt, 2007). Interpretation, in this context, has been pinpointed as the standard procedure for this purpose (Beuving & de Vries, 2015; Creswell, 2007). In his *Dictionary of Qualitative Inquiry*, Thomas Schwandt (2007, p. 158, emphasis added) defines interpretation as 'the act of clarifying, explicating, or explaining *the meaning* of some phenomenon'. Meaning is always at the centre of qualitative research.

Psychoanalytic interpretation acknowledges the importance of everyday language, and especially the actual words expressed in human interactions, yet it begins by suspending the privilege of meaning (Hook, 2013; Neill, 2013; Nobus & Quinn, 2005; Pavón-Cuéllar, 2014). This is what Lacan (1991, p. 73) had in mind when he advanced the somewhat disconcerting idea that, when it comes to interpretation, 'it is on the basis of a kind of refusal of understanding that we push open the door to analytic understanding'. Such is the quandary of Lacanian-informed social research: the deployment of qualitative methods to pursue a goal that runs counter to the principles of standard qualitative enquiry. Language is key not because it serves as a conduit for meaningful action within a symbolic environment, but because our efforts to produce meaning through it reveal the articulation of unconscious desire. From a psychoanalytic perspective, this is the primary function of language. And this is also why the unconscious is not synonymous with a recondite, almost inaccessible reservoir of personhood. The unconscious is *a transindividual operation*—that part of the discourse 'which is not at the subject's disposal in reestablishing the continuity of his conscious discourse' (Lacan, 2006, p. 214). The unconscious becomes evident when we stumble upon the materiality of the signifier.

If there is one thing that Ross' exploration of the Paris Commune unequivocally demonstrates, it is that social change was not an aspirational goal or a future reward for the communards. Instead, in the symbolic practices organising their everyday life, 'emancipation *was already materially underway*' (Ross, 2024, p. 2). By drawing parallels with Ross' approach, I have sought to show, first, the consequences of this materiality from a Lacanian point of view and, second, a viable way of studying it in the context of the Chilean revolt. As I explained earlier, there is no template for grasping the materiality of the signifier, only principles we must adhere to. As Lacan (1998, p. 33) puts it: 'The status of the unconscious, which, as I have shown, is so fragile on the ontic plane, is ethical. In his thirst for truth, Freud says, *Whatever it is, I must go there*, because, somewhere, this unconscious reveals itself'. So long as we rely on language to transmit the meaning of the *estallido*, our speech will articulate the desire for social change regardless of our conscious intention. The ethical decision is whether or not we pay attention to what it says. Guided by the psychoanalytic principles I have outlined in this chapter, I went there and diligently waited for those fragile expressions of the rebelliousness of the unconscious to reveal themselves. And they *reveal themselves* because desire is 'like being told a secret about oneself that someone else has made. It could never be a confession, because the confessor always already knows his secrets' (Phillips, 2006, p. 43). The secrets about the critical scholars made by the Other of the revolt constitute the delicate existence I tried to capture in the materiality of their speech.

References

Aedo, A., Bernasconi, O., Martínez, D., Olivari, A., Pairican, F., & Porma, J. (2024). Multitude and Memory in the Chilean Social Uprising. *The South Atlantic Quarterly, 123*(1), 192–202.

Bernes, J. (2025). *The Future of Revolution: Communist Prospects from the Paris Commune to the George Floyd Uprising*. Verso.

Beuving, J., & de Vries, G. (2015). *Doing Qualitative Research: The Craft of Naturalistic Inquiry*. Amsterdam University Press.

Castillo, A. (2019). *Asamblea de los Cuerpos*. Sangría Editora.

Copjec, J. (2015). *Read my Desire*. Verso.

Creswell, J. (2007). *Qualitative Inquiry & Research Design*. SAGE Publications.

Critchley, S. (2008). *Infinitely Demanding: Ethics of Commitment*. Verso.

Dardot, P. (2023). *La Memoria del Futuro, Chile 2019–2022*. Editorial Gedisa.

Dean, J. (2025). *Capital's Grave*. Verso.

Denzin, N., & Lincoln, Y. (2005). Introduction: The Discipline and Practice of Qualitative Research. In N. Denzin & Y. Lincoln (Eds.), *The SAGE Handbook of Qualitative Research*. SAGE Publications.

Edelman, L. (2004). *No Future: Queer Theory and the Death Drive*. Duke University Press.

Freud, S. (2001). Introductory Lectures on Psycho-analysis (1916–1917[1915–1917]). In *The Standard Edition of the Complete Psychological Works of Sigmund Freud, Vol. XV (1915–1916)*. Vintage.

Garretón, M. A. (2015). La recomposición de la triple vocación de la ciencia social en América Latina. *Polis, 14*(41), 159–173.

Glynos, J. (2021). Critical Fantasy Studies. *Journal of Language and Politics, 20*(1), 95–111.

Heyes, C. (2011). Subjectivity and Power. In D. Taylor (Ed.), *Michel Foucault: Key Concepts*. Acumen.

Hook, D. (2013). Tracking the Lacanian Unconscious in Language. *Psychodynamic Practice, 19*(1), 38–54.

Kaufman, E. (2020). Surface Critique: Althusser, Foucault, and the Problem of Ricardo. *The South Atlantic Quarterly, 119*(4), 747–759.

Kornbluh, A. (2014). *Realizing Capital: Financial and Psychic Economies in Victorian Form*. Fordham University Press.

Lacan, J. (1991). *The Seminar of Jacques Lacan, Book I: Freud's Papers on Technique*. W. W. Norton & Company.

Lacan, J. (1997a). *The Seminar of Jacques Lacan, Book III: The Psychoses, 1955–1956*. W. W. Norton & Company.
Lacan, J. (1997b). *The Seminar of Jacques Lacan, Book VII: The Ethics of Psychoanalysis*. W. W. Norton & Company.
Lacan, J. (1998). *The Seminar of Jacques Lacan, Book XI: The Four Fundamental Concepts of Psychoanalysis*. W. W. Norton & Company.
Lacan, J. (2006). The Function and Field of Speech and Language in Psychoanalysis. In *Écrits: The First Complete Edition in English*. W. W. Norton & Company.
Lacan, J. (2007). *The Seminar of Jacques Lacan, Book XVII: The Other Side of Psychoanalysis*. W. W. Norton & Company.
Lacan, J. (2008). *My Teaching*. Verso.
Lacan, J. (2019). *The Seminar of Jacques Lacan, Book VI: Desire and its Interpretation*. Polity.
Lacan, J. (2020). *The Seminar of Jacques Lacan, Book IV: The Object Relation*. Polity.
Lapping, C. (2016). Reflexivity and Fantasy: Surprising Encounters from Interpretation to Interruption. *Qualitative Inquiry, 22*(9), 718–724.
Lapping, C., & Glynos, J. (2018). Psychical Contexts of Subjectivity and Performative Practices of Remuneration: Teaching Assistants' Narratives of Work. *Journal of Education Policy, 33*(1), 23–42.
Leavy, P. (2014). Introduction. In P. Leavy (Ed.), *The Oxford Handbook of Qualitative Research*. Oxford University Press.
Martuccelli, D. (2021). *El Estallido Social en Clave Latinoamericana: La Formación de las Clases Popular-Intermediarias*. LOM Ediciones.
McGowan, T. (2016). *Capitalism and Desire: The Psychic Cost of Free Markets*. Columbia University Press.
McGowan, T. (2024). *Embracing Alienation: Why We Shouldn't Try to Find Ourselves*. Repeater Books.
Neill, C. (2013). Breaking the Text: An introduction to Lacanian Discourse Analysis. *Theory & Psychology, 23*(3), 334–350.
Nobus, D., & Quinn, M. (2005). *Knowing Nothing, Staying Stupid: Elements for a Psychoanalytic Epistemology*. Routledge.
Pavón-Cuéllar, D. (2014). From the Word to the Event: Limits, Possibilities and Challenges of Lacanian Discourse Analysis. In I. Parker & D. Pavón-Cuéllar (Eds.), *Lacan, Discourse, Event: New Psychoanalytic Approaches to Textual Indeterminacy*. Routledge.
Phillips, A. (2006). Desiring by Myself. In J. Petrucelli (Ed.), *Longing: Psychoanalytic Musings on Desire*. Karnac Books.

Phillips, A. (2018). Looking at Obstacles. In *One Way and Another: New and Selected Essays*. Penguin.

Puga, I. (2020). Ideological Inversion and the (de)legitimation of Neoliberalism in Chile. In X. Bada & L. Rivera-Sánchez (Eds.), *The Oxford Handbook of the Sociology of Latin America*. Oxford University Press.

Ross, K. (2016). *Communal Luxury: The Political Imaginary of the Paris Commune*. Verso.

Ross, K. (2023). *The Politics and Poetics of Everyday Life*. Verso.

Ross, K. (2024). *The Commune Form: The Transformation of Everyday Life*. Verso.

Schwandt, T. (2007). *The SAGE Dictionary of Qualitative Inquiry*. SAGE Publications.

Woods, M. (2022). *On the Chilean Social Explosion*. Routledge.

Žižek, S. (1997). *The Plague of Fantasies*. Verso.

Žižek, S. (2008). *The Sublime Object of Ideology*. Verso.

Žižek, S. (2000). Class Struggle or Postmodernism? Yes, Please! In J. Butler, E. Laclau, & S. Žižek (Eds.), *Contingency, Hegemony, Universality: Contemporary Dialogues on the Left*. Verso.

3
The Fantasy of Sleeplessness

In this chapter, I begin my interpretation of the responses to the desiring call of the Other in the *estallido*. My analysis focuses on an activity that appears ostensibly straightforward and simple: seeing the popular uprising unfold. In many ways, not seeing it was a practical challenge, as its presence could be felt wherever one looked. The revolt was characterised by the production of a rich, almost baroque visual landscape that saturated eyes and screens to an unprecedented scale in Chile. Despite how unavoidable it was to observe the revolt, the argument of this chapter is that the act of seeing entailed a range of ambivalent psychic dynamics. To perceive this, the first step is to suspend the apparent naturalness of the visual field. The Chilean writer Lina Meruane, who will make several appearances in this chapter, offers an illustration of this. She wrote an essay in which she encapsulates a generalised feeling about the revolt, namely, that it allowed us 'to see like we have never seen before' (Meruane, 2021, p. 17). The metaphorical link between seeing and the recognition of the oppressive organisation of life is clear, but what *exactly*

An abridged version of this chapter was published in *Psychoanalysis, Culture & Society, 29*(3), 2024.

G. Sánchez, *A Rebel Unconscious*, Studies in the Psychosocial,
https://doi.org/10.1007/978-3-032-12275-9_3

made it feel as though we were seeing completely anew? If the *estallido* did not eradicate neoliberalism but instead allowed us to experience it according to the logic of post-neoliberalism, then it is this new symbolic environment that turned seeing into a wholly novel experience.

The above suggests that the act of seeing and the symbolic are far more proximate than they may appear at first glance. As Joan Copjec (2015, p. 34) puts it, there is no such thing as a 'brute vision', since a vision 'totally independent of language' cannot be found. This means that the visual field is not given in advance but is symbolically organised. My interpretation will evince that this is not equivalent to saying that the order of things is historically determined by power relations, such that we cannot but see from a particular position. The fact that the revolt enabled us to see as we had never seen before indicates that we do not look at things with our eyes but with our desire. Or, which amounts to the same, that our vision is inextricably related to the Other and its (lack of) recognition. Lacanian psychoanalysis thus rejects the idea that visual reality is the 'background against which and in which we desire', and instead assumes it 'as a field thoroughly colored by our desire' (McGowan, 2016, p. 87). This implies that, to use a technical term, in the scopic field of the revolt the subject faces the enigma of the desire of the Other. This link between the visual and the symbolic explains why the unconscious effects of the call of the Other can be grasped in the act of seeing.

The visual richness of the Chilean revolt has been the focus of several studies (Badilla & Aguilera, 2021; De Vivanco & Johansson, 2021; Grimmer, 2025; Márquez, 2020; Pinochet, 2021). This is the case because the *estallido* brought about a wide range of artistic expressions that saturated its scopic field. Simultaneously, however, the revolt was marked by extreme cases of police misconduct that resulted in hundreds of protesters being totally or partially blinded. My interpretation touches on both these extremes of the popular uprising, yet I emphasise the unconscious dynamics at play in seeking recognition from the Other. In this sense, it has been suggested that protesters populated the streets amid a profound sense of equality, perceiving themselves as someone 'who has something to say and show, and who hopes to be recognised' (López, 2021, p. 20). The fact that recognition was at stake in the visual field of the revolt means that subjects were confronted with the gaze of the Other of the *estallido*, which can only result in misrecognition.

In the rest of this chapter, I reconstruct what I call the fantasy of sleeplessness. This is an imaginary framework that allowed critical academics to unconsciously endure the misrecognition they received from the Other by framing their desire. In particular, this fantasy emerges as the unconscious flipside of the main motto of the revolt: 'Chile woke up'. This phrase, 'the first big cry of the revolt' (Fernández, 2020, p. 15), set in motion a narrative based on the idea of a nationwide awakening after long decades of neoliberal somnolence. The very act of seeing thus became a way of recognising oneself within a post-neoliberal experience. The fantasy of sleeplessness was one of the ways in which this was unconsciously registered by concealing the participation of the subject in what it sees. This is what Lacanian psychoanalysis refers to as the split between the eye and the gaze: inasmuch as a passage through the signifier is inescapable for us to see, desire inevitably distorts the visual field, so we must obfuscate our implication in what we see. Therefore, the eye itself is phallic (Frosh, 2013), meaning that it is the guarantor of an imaginary stabilisation of the visible, whereas the gaze is the imprint of our desire returned to us from the outside—yet it remains beyond our capacity to register it consciously. These ideas will help us understand the unconscious effects of being called as someone who has awakened during the *estallido.*

The Revolt's New Eyes: Chile Woke Up

> burst [*estallido*]
> It was happening. Right then, happening. They'd been warning me for a long time, and yet. I was paralyzed, my sweaty hands clutching at the air [...]. And then a firecracker went off in my head. But no, it was no fire I was seeing, it was blood spilling out inside my eye. The most shockingly beautiful blood I have ever seen. The most outrageous. The most terrifying. The blood gushed, but only I could see it. With absolute clarity I watched as it thickened, I saw the pressure rise, I watched as I

> got dizzy, I saw my stomach turn, saw that I was starting to retch, and even so. I didn't straighten up or move an inch, didn't even try to breathe while I watched the show. Because that was the last thing I would see, that night, through that eye: a deep, black blood.
>
> *
>
> When I saw him arrive, I knew that he had to be my priority. He came in without his eyes. Tears of blood ran down his cheeks, and he couldn't speak because of the shock. I have experience in tragedies; I was in Chañaral looking for missing people [after the flooding], I was in the eruption of the Melipeuco volcano, and I worked in the Concepción earthquake. But this was completely out of the ordinary – I had never seen damage of this magnitude, let alone visual damage. It was all very shocking.

Despite their similarities, these excerpts come from different sources. The first is how *Seeing Red*, by Lina Meruane (2017, pp. 3–4), begins. The novel, published in 2012, is a fictionalised autobiography revolving around the vicissitudes of Lucinda, a Chilean author diagnosed with retinopathy, following an internal haemorrhage that left her almost totally blind. The second is the testimony of José González, a nurse member of The Brigade, a group of 45 health workers organised to assist protesters in downtown Santiago in the wake of the *estallido*. What José describes in the quotation is his encounter with Gustavo Gatica, a 21-year-old demonstrator who has become one of the most emblematic cases of police brutality during the revolt. He lost both eyes as a result of being hit by 'non-lethal' shells fired by the police. Gustavo, however, was by no means an exception, yet I shall return to this shortly. In the interim, I would like to emphasise how Meruane's book, in retrospect, appears to be an eerie omen: in 2012, she was writing about another *estallido*, that of her eye; seven years later, this would become an ignominious feature of our own social *estallido*. Seeing during the revolt, as this chapter will show, was nothing short of a novel experience.

Eyes have been at the centre of the *estallido* since the beginning. Some were taken by police ammunition, some were irritated by tear gas, but, on the whole, all of them were finally opened—at least this is what the motto 'Chile woke up' suggests. After realising his sight was irretrievably gone, Gustavo Gatica said to his mother: 'I gave away my eyes so that people wake up'. Now that a few years have passed since this sentence was uttered, breaking it down seems less callous than it might have while the events were still unfolding. On the one hand, Gustavo's phrase almost seems to be extracted from a novel. Lines as inspiring as the one he delivered from his stretcher are rarely pronounced in everyday life, let alone in his condition. The aplomb and composure he exhibited in the face of a life-changing situation surely account for the emboldening effect his words had among protesters, as he urged them to keep fighting. On the other hand, this is an excellent example of how meaning is always a retroactive and imaginary construction. Once the *estallido* was framed under the heading 'Chile woke up', the abuse of power he was subjected to was transformed into a kind of gift—an oblation to the cause of bringing the country out of its dormancy. Outside this overarching narrative, losing your eyes due to police brutality can hardly be considered an offering. But Chile, as many felt, had woken up.

'Chile woke up' was everywhere, and it was just about anything—a chant on the streets, an amorphous collective feeling, the headline of many news articles, a catchphrase on innumerable banners, the inspiration for a range of performances, the title of several academic papers and books, and even the name of an art tour around the streets of Santiago. For months, the idea that Chile was no longer asleep was almost unquestionable and everybody had a take on what that could mean. In a way, as Gustavo Gatica embodies in all its woeful complexity, waking up was the encouraging reverse of the harrowing numbers of mutilated eyes. The unparalleled scale in which eyes were 'lost' in Chile allowed human rights watchdogs to call it an 'epidemic' (United Nations, 2019), while Meruane (2021, p. 34) coined the idea of a 'serial eye-cide'. In Chile, hundreds of eyes were temporarily or permanently blinded so millions of other eyelids would never come into contact again. And as easy as it may be to treat this hyperbolic statement as an embellishment or a metaphor for the situation, it nevertheless holds some literalness. 'Don't you ever fall asleep' was a graffiti I spotted every day while walking back to the house of a friend in Santiago, where I spent a good part of my fieldwork. This is important to stress: if the Chilean people were to honour the gift of Gustavo and many others, their unmutilated eyes must *never* close again. Or, as Meruane (2021, p. 17) once again wrote: 'OPEN

YOUR EYES. That order written on walls and façades full of half-open windows. We abide by the persuasive urgency'. She wrote that line almost three years after the revolt began. By then, according to her, this order had not yet lost its interpellative force.

Lorena, a PhD student, succinctly summarises the spirit of this nation-wide awakening: 'I went outside again but I was now looking at the streets differently, as in with other eyes'. There are at least two ways to approach this. We can either immerse ourselves in the discourse formation that renders such statements meaningful, namely, the idea that Chile actually woke up from something yet to be determined; or we can rehearse a suspension of this imaginary meaningfulness and remain at a symbolic level. From the first position, Lorena's 'other eyes' are an answer—they are straightforwardly the upshot of the revolt. From the second position, this new pair of eyes is more of a question; not so much a question of what they mean, but of what they represent within the libidinal economy of the revolt. Put differently, from a symbolic perspective, what comes to the fore are the associations that the 'other eyes' mobilise to recognise oneself as someone who has woken up. This is all the more pertinent when we bear in mind that, from a Lacanian stance, the gaze is never on the side of the subject, so in a way, we *always* look with other eyes. In consequence, 'eye, look and desire are all bound up together' (Frosh, 2013, p. 76). These somewhat cryptic ideas can lend us a hand in understanding the vicissitudes of the Other's call amid the *estallido*.

To pin down what the Chilean people might have woken up from is no simple task. The certainty of the awakening disproportionately outweighs the clarity surrounding the roots of the slumber. Neoliberalism, as is often the case, stands as the main culprit in most interviews, although this, in itself, is far from illuminating. For instance, Ramón—a member of the academic staff of a prestigious PhD programme—suggests that 'neoliberalism has made us very sleepy'; so, for him, something as disruptive as the *estallido* was close to unimaginable. Isabel, a scholar at one of the largest public universities in the country, also resorts to neoliberalism, albeit through an idiosyncratic proxy—the idea of 'the model'. In her view, the deepening of the neoliberal model over the thirty years that followed the dictatorship also exerted a soporific effect on Chileans. Her take, however, is far more ambivalent than Ramón's:

> We found in our research this relentless uneasiness with the transitional pact coming out in the stories of the post-dictatorship, you know? And I was amazed, prior to the *estallido*, amazed at how calm everything was; it seemed that deep down everyone had already settled in and they had no choice but to put up with it, you know? But we all knew, I mean, when I talked to people for my *fondecyt* [research grant], everyone, well, no, everyone on the left had a critical vision, right? A critical vision of what the *Concertación* governments had been, of what the [transitional] pact had been like, and so on. So, when the *estallido* occurred, we said: "well, now the common people have woken up".

As Chapter 7 will show in detail, *fondecyts*—those highly competitive and prestigious state-funded research projects—play a significant libidinal role in the fantasmatic scaffolding that sustains academic identities in Chile. I will postpone that discussion and focus here on the rest of the quotation. In a way, and despite identifying the same underlying cause, Isabel reaches the exact opposite conclusion to Ramón: when considering all the social discontent that had accumulated over three decades, the *estallido* seems entirely imaginable. Thanks to her research grant, she had first-hand knowledge of this growing disappointment concealed by a generalised appearance of calm. She knew how things stood, so, in a sense, it was only a matter of time before the common people followed suit.

There are two particularly relevant aspects of this line of thought that I would like to highlight. On the one hand, the lethargic powers of neoliberalism are, to some extent, counterintuitive. Chileans were not drifting off because their lives were uneventful, but because they were ceaselessly producing. Neoliberalism demands that people work 'from dawn to dusk', to continually do more and more—and that makes them drowsy. On the other hand, sleeping is linked to knowledge, or more precisely, to the lack thereof. This is conveyed not only through the discursive invocation of research grants, but especially in the more colloquial moments of our conversation. When Isabel went into further details about this unsettling calmness, she admitted: 'I said to myself many times, like these people are asle… they are thick, that was my expression (laughs): thick'. Although very hard to translate, the slur she uses harshly denotes a stupid, gullible person; it communicates the idea of a profound lack of understanding. As a result, the lapse in her self-censorship here is highly revealing: 'asleep' is a much more palatable term to describe this stupid other, who is affiliated with a group to which she clearly does not belong and, it is likely to infer, assumes I do not belong either. This might explain why she let her guard down, allowing herself to unbind a more discourteous association: being asleep = being thick.

We thus arrive at a minimal definition: to wake up is to have one's eyes open in order to know. The correlation between seeing clearly—having our eyes open/not being asleep—and knowledge has deep roots in the Western tradition. Ocularcentrism is the rather flamboyant name given to this epistemological ascendancy of vision over other senses. Although the conceptual relationship between seeing and knowing is indeed compelling in the context of the revolt (see San Martín et al., 2023), my interest lies in the symbolic associations produced by critical scholars in order to sustain this relationship. In this regard, the experience of Nicolás, a PhD researcher and part-time lecturer, is worthy of close attention. He engaged with the revolt not only at an academic level but also through creative practices, which made him particularly receptive to its visual dimensions.

Seeing Things as a Dream

I interviewed Nicolás twice during May 2022. On these occasions, I encountered someone deeply moved by the revolt—both in the sense of being emotionally affected by the events and in feeling compelled to recognise himself in the awakening. He found various practical avenues through which to navigate the latter, yet addressing the *estallido* was not an easy task for him. This can be perceived in the way he used the term 'dream' and the associations it evoked. One of these associations touches on an aspect often overlooked by some of my interviewees despite its omnipresence: the violence unleashed by the revolt. Nicolás introduces the notion of a 'time of catastrophe' to describe the final months of 2019.

'That time', he acknowledges, 'I see it as a dream'. The dreamlike experience he alludes to here relates to a sense of temporal unreliability—as normally happens in dreams, there is a vagueness regarding the temporality one inhabits. For him, 'the boundaries were extremely diffuse' at the time, meaning that what he describes as days could easily have been weeks or even months. Superimposed as they are, his reflections reveal a twofold relationship between dreaming and the time of catastrophe: under such conditions, real life begins to resemble certain aspects of dream life, but we also tend to dream more profoundly and vividly. The dreamlike chaos of the catastrophe renews our ties with the act of dreaming, 'as if the dream begins to reveal or to manifest itself through this uncertainty one's in during the day'.

At this early stage, it is already evident that we should refrain from understanding this 'dreaming' as an activity confined to our beds during the night. Nicolás appears to be expressing something significantly different. In the context of the catastrophe, he admits that 'there was a lot of tension, inside the house I mean, a tension that I now see as a dream'. He, once again, is seeing things *in the form of a dream*, yet he is not dreaming in any literal sense. This is an interesting use of the term. Nonetheless, the tension he recalls had very tangible manifestations. Pillaging was one of them. Nicolás' home was located within walking distance of the city centre, and just a few streets away stood a big supermarket that 'got bulldozed day and night' in a plundering spree that continued for days. Another manifestation was the curfew. Imposed by the chief of the National Defence almost immediately in the capital and subsequently extended to other cities, it marked the first time this measure had been enforced for political reasons since the dictatorship. 'The curfew', Nicolás continues, 'that shit was unthinkable; I honestly can't believe it'. For him, the idea of going out to stock up on food and other essentials only to return and lock oneself in was absurd: 'It was surreal, you know? It was like a dream, like a nightmare'.

Up to this point, the term 'dream' has been mobilised to convey a sense of a temporal unreliability, a revelation, a tension, and the unthinkable (a nightmare). What these usages have in common is their connection to various manifestations of the *estallido*, though not to the event as such. This changes when Nicolás begins to speak about his work and, crucially, the work of others. Quite suddenly, his tone acquires a bitterness hitherto unexpressed, directed at certain artists he considers 'political'. Some artists, he claims, took advantage of the unfolding situation to quickly and opportunistically produce images that allowed them to feel 'proper', as if they 'truly belong to the streets'. At this point, he takes aim at what is perhaps the most iconic artistic expression of the revolt:

> Take the DelightLab. They projected the images on the Telefónica building and like, well, they took to it like a duck to water, you know? They're like, they're doing amazing, and they're being invited everywhere because they generated an image of the *estallido*, right? But like, like I think the *estallido* is similar to a dream, because it's uncapturable, you know? So that uncapturable, wanting to give it an image, for me is extremely irresponsible; for me, wanting to reduce it to a definition is irresponsible.

DelightLab is an art collective that has been experimenting with light and space for over a decade in Chile. The day after the revolt began, they decided to project several words and short phrases each day onto the Telefónica building, a 143-metre-high skyscraper adjacent to Dignity Square.[1] Among their interventions, they illuminated the city with the phrase 'Chile woke up'. In one of the many interviews given by its members, the collective aligned itself with an activist, political form of art, referring to their work as a 'luminous manifesto'. Their light-based activism has since become the focus of several studies, which tend to underscore that, due to 'the immediacy of their digital circulation', these images helped 'resist dominant narratives and articulate new collective meanings' (Pinochet, 2021, p. 549; see also Grimmer, 2025). Yet this does not sit well with Nicolás. Following the thread of his own speech, what troubles him is that they 'captured' the *estallido*; they treated it as an image rather than as a dream. In contrast to the image, Nicolás articulates rich symbolic associations through his singular relationship

[1] Like almost every other revolt during the mass protest decade (Bevins, 2023), Santiago's main square—officially named 'Baquedano' after a military general—was anonymously rechristened as 'Dignity Square' during the *estallido*. For an insightful discussion of the affinities between contemporary forms of assembly and spatial configuration, see Müller (2024).

with dreaming. What he discursively constructs is the antagonistic figure of an opportunistic other, a figure that moves along the axis 'image = capturable = irresponsibility', as opposed to 'dream = uncapturable = responsibility'. What 'dream' stands for, however, remains unspecified.

Nicolás gives me a hint of the above when he explains in more detail why he adopts a combative stance towards political art. To begin with, he clarifies that he is not hostile to politically inspired art. On the contrary, what he takes issue with is 'the political art that's called "political art" because it talks about politics, and it seems that other things aren't'. From his perspective, the kind of art that directly registers the political as a sort of conveyor belt of events does a disservice to the cause from which these events emerge. Returning to the *estallido*, to merely replicate through an image that 'Chile woke up' seems, for Nicolás, to benefit the artist alone, at the expense of diminishing the political capacity of art. At this point, Nicolás begins to vociferate: 'They make it look as if the relationship with your son, with your daughter, with your partner, with your friends, that shit ain't political, right? Or what you dreamed last night ain't political, right?' The irresponsibility, then, of turning a dream into an image lies in the foreclosure of its political potentialities.

While still conveying his ideas in an oppositional fashion, his speech begins to link the dream to more positive terms. For him, addressing the revolt should be 'like starting to associate things from a place that has no associativity whatsoever', or 'to talk about things without talking about them'. What this procedure avoids, in Nicolás' view, is the propensity to fall prey to 'the reduction of the image, the narrowing of a definition'. Adopting his own idiom, what he wants is to 'beat around the bush endlessly'. At a key point in his speech, he goes over the reasons for his deep interest in dreams:

> And why dreams? Well, because my auntie healed through distance, in the vigil; it is as though she visited you (laughs). Like: "I'm gonna go to heal you, I'm gonna go to see you in the night". So, for me, she healed through dreams and, after talking with her – she passed away a couple of years ago – she told me: "yeah, I dream, you know? I dream that I'm gonna see you", and that stuck with me.

The richness of this short excerpt is exceptional. Some background information is required first. The precise genealogy of the unorthodox therapy Nicolás refers to is beyond my grasp, but suffice it to say that I myself grew up in an environment where the idea of someone visiting you in your dreams to heal an ailment is nothing out of the ordinary. My mother is, in this regard, the most reliable academic source. She swears by an entire constellation of treatments derived from what she calls 'ancient wisdom'. There are several expressions of this: tying a red ribbon to a plant or a baby's wrist to repel the evil eye; picking bits of skin around the spine of someone who feels unwell to 'unstick' whatever they have attached to the stomach; or setting fire to cones made of newspaper sheets and wafting them over the body of someone suffering from 'trapped air'. Dream visitations sit at the upper echelons of this wisdom—something that only certain women can achieve. It is conventionally a form of knowledge passed down from generation to generation. According to my mother, some of our neighbours were capable of this. In a different location, Nicolás' aunt was another one.[2]

Thanks to his aunt, we have arrived at a new association: dream = healing. This curative capacity, however, is not an intrinsic property of the dream—it is contingent on a visitant. Properly speaking, the dream operates here as a vehicle; it is the conduit for healing. Perhaps unwittingly, Nicolás makes a subsequent equivalence: he first says 'my auntie heals through distance', followed by 'she heals through dreams'. Healing through dreams *is* healing through distance. The dream, therefore, is an interval or a gap, an indirect way of doing something. Interestingly, this sanative capacity of the dream does not take place while both parties are asleep, but during the vigil, that is to say, *in a forced state of wakefulness*. Once again, this 'dream' has nothing to do with what happens when we

[2] It seems to me a matter of intellectual integrity, and an important methodological point, to acknowledge my transference with Nicolás. By this, I mean that sustaining my role as a researcher interviewing a participant of my study was, at times, very challenging. This is, of course, an imaginary setting that never works flawlessly, since shifting from one identification to another during the conversation is entirely normal (Lapping, 2011). However, both the relatability of his political positions and the unexpected shared experience of a sort of pagan knowledge running in our families made my job especially difficult. In a way, I had to keep reminding myself that the reason I was sitting in front of him was to follow his associations, not to get lost in them. During the interpretation of my material, much of this transference faded, due to a rather reasonable de-idealisation that emerged throughout the process.

are tucked up in bed. A brief etymological detour seems propitious here. *Visitar* ['to visit']—the verb used by Nicolás when describing his auntie's technique—comes from the Latin *visitāre*, which in turn means 'to go to see'. Quite literally, then, what happens for Nicolás is that the dream *sees him* in the night, and he must be awake if he wants to be healed.

Nicolás was one of the kindest people I had the opportunity to interview, generous enough to share with me some personal writing about this very topic (a document that, for obvious reasons of anonymity, I will not reference in detail). There, for instance, I discovered that his auntie's knowledge was bestowed upon her by her mother, a woman who also had a significant impact on Nicolás' approach to dreams. She passed away when he was still a child, and somewhere in the text he describes how difficult it was to fall asleep afterwards: 'Night after night, I felt this calling, an abyss when the light was off; then, I recognised myself minuscule and I couldn't resist it anymore. The dream took hold of me and revealed its mysteries to me'. This passage bears a striking resemblance to Meruane's description of the injunction to stay awake after the revolt, quoted earlier. They both refer to a kind of interpellative capacity—the calling of the dream for him, the order of the revolt for her. For Nicolás, the dream was sanatory: it allowed him to respond to the call and cease to recognise himself as minuscule.

Sleeping with Your Eyes Open

Sleeping implies a peculiar dynamic. Much like being in love, sleep requires as its precondition stumbling upon something, for we cannot do it directly; rather, we must *fall* asleep. For sleep to occur, we need to fall victim to our own deception. As Darian Leader (2019) proposes, although sleeping is undoubtedly an essential, even natural, aspect of life, the need to engage in a series of mental gymnastics to induce it is a uniquely human trait. Otherwise stated, only speaking beings must partake in a self-organised sham in order to sleep. The reason for this, Leader suggests, can be found in the incompatibility between sleep and the self. In everyday life, we are required to rehearse various identifications in order to carry out our activities, and the same applies when it comes to sleep: we need to identify with the position of the sleeper. This is why a trick, a fall, must be part of the dynamic—to sleep, it is necessary *to accept being duped*.

Falling asleep, from this perspective, entails bringing some of our daytime identifications to a halt. The Other's call must remain unanswered if we are to sleep.[3] This means not only ceasing to be a worker, a sibling, or a scholar, but crucially, momentarily setting aside the question of what the Other wants from us. This is what Nicolás finds himself unable to achieve. For as noble as it is to want to transform Chilean society, embracing the idea that 'Chile woke up' dramatically altered our relationship with sleep. My point here is not simply that, in a context where being awake is an order, as Meruane puts it, we suffer from a suspension of sleep. Rather, my interpretation is slightly more nuanced: one of the outcomes of the *estallido* is that we can no longer *fall* asleep. This is what Nicolás' experience shows. 'Chile woke up' means that any attempt to soften the interpellation from the Other is bound to fail, since being duped by any trick is now overruled—yet this is precisely what is crucial for humans to sleep. Finding recognition in the Other's wake-up call entails identifying with the position of a knower—an identification that cannot be broken, for otherwise, the experience of the end of neoliberalism falters. Finally, after a three-decade-long slumber, our eyes are wide open and only someone 'thick' would dare to close them again.

I would like to provide a succinct yet powerful illustration of the interpellative force of the revolt within the visual field. María is a PhD researcher whose work revolves around sex workers. The nature of her topic made her especially attentive to the visuality of the *estallido*; all of a sudden, as she notes, no group of people or identity was condemned to remain out of sight any longer. Other feminist researchers have also observed how the 'visual culture' of the revolt 'made visible and empowered female, dissident, and subaltern bodies. Streets, walls, buildings,

[3] Using a different language, Freud (2001a, p. 128) made the exact same point: 'we have forgotten that besides somatic stimuli there are *mental* stimuli that disturb sleep. We know, after all, that it is excitations of this kind that are chiefly responsible for disturbing the sleep of an adult by preventing him from establishing the mood required for falling asleep–the withdrawing of interest from the world. He does not want to interrupt his life but would rather continue his work on the things he is concerned with, and for that reason he does not fall asleep'.

and squares were transformed by the feminist rebellion that imagines an inclusive and plurinational order' (Llanos, 2021, p. 68). While this is undeniable, María also described how this transformation of the city's appearance could be perceived in the way 'the streets were yelling at you':

> In every street of Santiago one can see some slogan, some graffiti, you know? So, it is like a permanent visual reminder of the problem. Like I was on my way to the grocery store the other day and I glanced on the wall "Bobbies are rapists" [*pacos violadores*], you know? And I thought: "yeah, Bobbies do rape". And it is a very important reminder. I don't know, I went to the supermarket and [saw on the wall] "No more SENAME" [the public institution for the protection of children and adolescents], and you are there, so you remember there are some kiddos experiencing an inhumane situation within the system [...], so it helps you remember what the topics are... what the mottoes are; it helps you to, they help you to... like, unexpectedly, without you wanting to, you walk down the street and you read a slogan, you know? "Free political prisoners", and you could ask yourself, I insist, while walking the dog, "are there political prisoners?", "who are the political prisoners?" So there, visually, there are stimuli that weren't there before, right?

It is hard to find a more eloquent description of the call of the Other during the revolt: the relentless, unexpected, and insidious *visual reminder* that you *must know*—even 'without you wanting to'. Chile woke up, and an unquenchable interpellative force was unleashed in the form of a ceaseless self-doubt: I am walking my dog, but should I instead be thinking about misogyny in the police force, our non-existent social security services, and political prisoners? Do I know? Or am I awake? If we are, then we must witness everything; no one can ever fall asleep. Paradoxically, this way of securing identification with the revolt seems structurally analogous to the previous position: neoliberalism made Chileans drowsy through the demand for endless productivity, and the revolt kept them awake by means of an interminable self-questioning. Even if the latter seeks to reverse the former, both share the same fundamental logic: an unstoppable activity. While the endless neoliberal movement had a stultifying effect on Chileans, the *estallido* set in motion an emancipatory counterattack rooted in an unfaltering state of inquisitive wonder. Either in the form of neoliberalism or of revolt, the call of the Other knows no boundary.

What, then, is *seeing things as a dream*? Following the interpretation I have presented here, it is Nicolás' fantasmatic solution to the problem of *falling* asleep during the revolt. In other words, it is an unconscious way of *sleeping with his eyes open*—of imaginarily disengaging without betraying the imperative to remain alert. At several moments in his speech, he adopts a rather overzealous position on how people ought to treat the *estallido*. The latter should not be 'captured', 'defined', or 'put in images'; it should be treated 'responsibly'. By wanting to 'talk about it without talking about it' or to 'establish associations without any associativity', Nicolás assumes that the only legitimate way of approaching the revolt is by establishing a purely contemplative distance. A distance akin to the one his auntie resorted to in order to heal him—the distance of the dream, we might say.

Nicolás appears here to take the *estallido* to the letter: if he gets too close to it, he shall combust. The flames, nevertheless, are nearby, lurking, since they have taken the shape of a burning interpellation coming from every corner. Interestingly, at this point we can perceive that Nicolás' fantasy is not so much an attempt to respond to the Other's call as it is an effort to identify with the Other itself. He is acutely aware that being duped is no longer permitted—that he must know about everything—and that is why he proceeds so cautiously; he dreads closing his eyes and being caught in the mistake. Confronted with the impossibility of either responding to or evading the call that the Other of the *estallido* directs to him, he fantasises about *seeing* with the eyes of the Other—the only eyes that are not duped—in order to escape its omniscient sight. His unconscious desire is to see from a safe place: the Other's sanatory distance. This is the imaginary place where he can psychically tolerate the call of the Other—where he can drift off without the fall, without the trick, and, ultimately, without surrendering to the vulnerability that sleep requires.

Within Nicolás' speech, the signifier 'dream' organises a libidinally charged scenario in which it is fantasmatically possible to deal with this demanding Other by identifying with it. Accordingly, this imaginary sleepless setting is erected upon a fantasy of *pure interpellation*. Inasmuch as the call of the Other of the *estallido* is unanswerable—since the revolt made of the fictional, properly 'tricky' wrapping of our social interactions its main adversary—Nicolás finds a measure of tranquillity in sublimating the dream as a site of unconscious investment. This solution is, of course, not without ambivalence. Insomniacs, Leader (2019) argues, are those who cannot turn the interpellation off; those for whom silencing the question of what they are for the Other proves to be unobtainable. However, he also suggests that sleeplessness can spring from something even worse: the tormenting thought that there is nothing calling us at all. This dialectic lies at the heart of Nicolás' fantasy. *Seeing as a dream* is a way of imaginarily escaping from interpellation by perpetuating it—Nicolás allows himself to *fall* asleep, to switch off the call of the Other, by enthroning himself as the custodian of this interpellation. Consequently, this fantasmatic construction shows us how difficult it is to cope with the burning call of the revolt but, simultaneously, that the idea of not being called by it might be even harder to psychically endure.

One of the most famous dreams in psychoanalytic literature is 'the burning child'. An exhausted father who 'had been watching beside his child's sick-bed for days and nights on end', decides to go to rest in the next room, leaving the door open 'so that he could see from his bedroom into the room in which his child's body was laid out'. An old man remains behind with the mandate to watch over the body in the father's absence, murmuring prayers. The father falls asleep and dreams 'that *his child was standing beside his bed, caught him by the arm and whispered to him reproachfully: "Father, don't you see I'm burning?"*' (Freud, 2001b, p. 509). He wakes up to discover that the old watchman has also fallen asleep and that one of the arms of his dead child has been caught by the flames of the candles. The richness of this dream has captivated many commentators. The incisive reading of Cathy Caruth (1996) provides important insights into Nicolás' experience.

Caruth notes that Freud and Lacan approached this dream with different questions in mind. Whereas Freud argues that the dream keeps the father asleep—since within the oneiric world he fulfils the desire of seeing his child alive—Lacan claims that, paradoxically, the father wakes up precisely because he dreams. This counterintuitive reading points to the fact that, for Lacan, the father is awakened not by the fall of the candle, but by the words he could only receive in the form of a dream. As a result, while Freud asks what it means to sleep, Lacan instead poses the question of what it means to awaken. Caruth's interpretation is that, following Lacan, awakening is in itself traumatic. She defines trauma as 'the response to an unexpected or overwhelming violent event or events that are not fully grasped as they occur, but return later in repeated flashbacks, nightmares, and other repetitive phenomena' (Caruth, 1996, p. 91). The trauma of awakening is related to the simultaneous necessity and impossibility of responding to someone's call. In Freud's dream, the father is addressed with words that reiterate both the need and impossibility of confronting the death of his child. Accordingly, she maintains that:

> From this perspective, the trauma that the dream, as an awakening, reenacts is not only the missed encounter with the child's death but also the way in which that missing also constitutes the very survival of the father. His survival must no longer be understood, in other words, merely as an accidental living beyond the child, but rather as a mode of existence determined by the impossible structure of the response. (Caruth, 1996, p. 100)

The words in the dream re-enact a missed encounter. This missed encounter is not that the father fails to see that his child is burning, but that he *fails to see it in time*. As Caruth puts it, what this interpretation demonstrates is that we are always addressed either too early or too late, but never at the right time. Consequently, we must rehearse a mode of existence grounded in the idea that a missed call is the only possible call from the Other. Returning to Nicolás, this is precisely what his 'dream' cannot integrate, what allows him to fantasmatically resist. His libidinal investment in this signifier appears to be a way of imaginarily avoiding the trauma of the revolt's call by assuming only its impossibility but not its necessity. Confronted with an impossible yet necessary interpellation, he identifies with the Other in an attempt to regain a safe recognition. This unconscious move, however, re-enacts the missed encounter. Thus, seeing things as a dream becomes Nicolás' way of sheltering himself from the real trauma of awakening.

What Did We Wake Up to?

The fantasy of sleeplessness can be read as the unconscious flipside of the revolt's motto 'Chile woke up'. The liberating impulse springing from the *estallido* coalesced symbolically around one of the most emblematic critical procedures, namely, the capacity to see how things really are behind the veil of ideology. As a result of the revolt, or so the narrative goes, Chileans were no longer under the soporific effects of the various expressions of neoliberal oppression. The *estallido*, then, is largely regarded as a collective awakening from subjugation. However, this emancipatory 'invitation' to identify as an awakened subject was also experienced as a disproportionate demand. Although indubitably metaphoric in intention, the idea of waking up came to imply a mandate: never to fall asleep ever again. Yet being awake and not sleeping are very different in nature. So, in order to sustain the redemptive aspect of the revolt, a very literal yet unconscious refusal to *fall* asleep emerged. One of the results was a fatigued subject who must go to great imaginary lengths to find some rest within a context in which falling asleep is equated with being duped.[4] I will suggest that the fantasy of sleeplessness can be more thoroughly understood as the response to a paradigmatically hallucinatory dimension of the motto 'Chile woke up'.

Commonly, hallucinations are defined as erroneous perceptions; more precisely, as perceptions without objects. For various reasons, we are capable of seeing things that simply are not there, a feature largely associated with psychoses. The psychoanalytic tradition, however, has broken with the stubborn idea that hallucinations are inherently abnormal phenomena. By way of example, Wilfred Bion distinguished between sane and insane psychotics, while Donald Winnicott maintained that

[4] This echoes the testimony of insomniacs. As Marie Darrieussecq (2023, p. 129) acknowledges: 'I don't know any lazy insomniacs. I only know exhausted insomniacs. Insomniacs stay in bed in order to sleep, and don't sleep. They are desperately in search of sleep time, time that is always lost'.

hallucinations are not an illness but a characteristic of the process of dream formation (Rose, 2004). Taking a step further in this direction, Lacan fully uncoupled his theory of hallucinations from the premise of erroneous perception.[5] The inaccuracy or unreality of hallucinatory perception is, in this view, entirely beside the point; what actually matters is its subjective effect. Hallucinations belong to the register of interpellation and allude to the Other, 'a term that is invariably present but never seen and never named except indirectly' (Lacan, 1997, p. 256). Following Stijn Vanheule (2011), from a Lacanian perspective hallucinations constitute an impasse with the Other in the form of an interruption in signification. Certain events, on account of their radical strangeness in relation to a given system of meaning, are impossible to integrate into the subject's experiential continuity. Hallucinations, then, point to this inconsistency in our identifications, insofar as the subject does not coincide with the hallucination but is, instead, subjected to it.

Based on this non-pathological conceptualisation of hallucinations, we can see that their substratum is not 'reality' but words. One expression of this verbal process is the 'message phenomenon'. Since meaning is always a retroactive creation—as jokes illustrate, it is the punchline that backwardly stabilises a sentence—incomplete or unfinished statements are indicative of interruptions in the process of meaning-making. In the case of message phenomena, this incompleteness is characterised by deferred punctuation: 'the interrupted sentence fails to convey a message but a movement of anticipating meaning is established [...], this interruption leads to a situation of enigma and suspension for the subject' (Vanheule, 2011, p. 97). Put differently, identifications cannot be sustained amid unfinished sentences, and this precipitates a hastiness in the subject to recalibrate its relationship with the Other. 'Chile woke up' stands as a primary example of deferred punctuation. Even if we accept that the country was indeed brought out of its dormancy by the revolt, it remains entirely unclear what Chile woke up *to*.

---

[5] 'Hallucinations are phenomena structured at the level of signifiers. One cannot, not even for an instant, think about the organization of these hallucinations without seeing that the first thing to be emphasized in the phenomenon is that it's a phenomenon of signifiers' (Lacan, 2017, p. 204).

In this precise and circumscribed sense, it can be said that the fantasy of sleeplessness hints at a hallucinatory dimension of the *estallido*. Once the latter begins to function as the Other, the point of reference for an emancipatory call, certain subjective challenges arise. Through the motto 'Chile woke up', the Other of the revolt offered the grounds for experiencing the end of neoliberalism but placed the responsibility for cushioning whatever that meant upon the subject's shoulders. This is its unfinished or deferred facet. Accordingly, the unconscious effects of 'Chile woke up' can be interpreted as hallucinatory insofar as the *estallido* gives rise to an unchained signifier that leaves the subject forlorn in the search for meaning. To the extent that Chile simply woke up but never woke up *to* anything in particular, the relationship between the subject and the Other became particularly problematic: the emancipatory invitation to recognise oneself as an awakened subject was imbued with misrecognition. Nicolás' fantasy was a way of navigating this situation.

The missing 'to', the unchained signifier in the narrative of the national awakening, further illuminates the singular relationship with the Other in the fantasy of sleeplessness. The metaphorical embellishment of the idea of never falling asleep again acquires an unconscious literalness precisely at the moment when the Other of the *estallido* is not there to punctuate its meaning. The result is an uninterrupted succession of possibilities that renders the revolt an unregistrable event in the subject's experience, to the point that any attempt to identify with it drifts without anchorage. Hence, the fantasy of sleeplessness is not so much a means of regaining a solid identification *with* the revolt as it is an unconscious mechanism for *avoiding* this traumatic call through a direct, yet impossible identification with the Other. 'Seeing things as a dream' is Nicolás' singular way of dodging the shortcomings of interpellation amid the *estallido* by imaginarily adopting the position of the Other, the place from which interpellation is launched. This is why his speech reproduces the logic of deferred punctuation when he speaks of the 'uncapturable' nature of the *estallido*—one that requires an 'association without associativity' or the act of 'talking without talking'. As a response to the Other sidestepping the 'to' in the formulation 'Chile woke up', Nicolás unconsciously circumvents the impossibility of falling asleep during the *estallido* by 'seeing' things as a dream.

By following the associations that the signifier 'dream' produced in Nicolás' speech, I have reconstructed a fantasmatic narrative that allows subjects to locate their unconscious desire and thus respond to the desiring call of the revolt. To identify as someone who lives neoliberalism according to the logic of post-neoliberalism, Chileans had to recognise themselves as those who had awakened. Nicolás' experience shows that this not a position we can occupy comfortably despite its conscious desirability, since '*there is no right moment to awaken*' (Žižek, 2023, p. 1). Particularly evident in the experience of those who self-bind to the good of post-neoliberalism, the process of finding oneself within the emancipatory wake-up call of the *estallido* was accompanied by an intense circuit of unconscious excess and antagonism. Among the peculiarities of this process, my interpretation suggests that, rather than solving problems, fantasies displace them. The more Nicolás talked about something seemingly as simple as looking, the more certain signifiers ceased to follow his conscious intention, revealing parallel associations that render 'seeing things as a dream' a problematic solution to the enigma of the revolt's desire.

From my interpretation it follows that the undoubtedly emancipatory motto 'Chile woke up' provoked intense subjective challenges among Chileans. Nicolás' speech attests to this, and his fantasy of sleeplessness constitutes an unconscious attempt to organise a possible solution. Torn between an exhausting interpellation and an equally distressing fear of not being the target of its call, it seems that, for him, one of the few unavoidable outcomes of the *estallido* is a subjective combustion. The revolt created the figure of an Other from whom nothing escapes its sight. In this context, the fight against neoliberal lethargy takes the form of endless daytime scrutiny. Nicolás identifies with the Other to appease this pressure, even at the cost of intensifying its grip. Ironically, what this emancipatory Other shares with the neoliberal, oppressive Other is a façade of solidity—as though they *really* can see everything. What both overlook is the fact that, as Copjec (2015, p. 36) reminds us, 'when you encounter the gaze of the Other, you meet not a seeing eye but a blind one'. Even if the Other is the site from which the emancipatory call is issued, this call does not reach the subject with the clarity of full vision but rather with the tentativeness of a groping gesture. Hence,

Nicolás' experience shows that even—or perhaps especially—in emancipatory settings, desire springs not from the success of the interpellative call, but from its failure.

References

Badilla, M., & Aguilera, C. (2021). The 2019–2020 Chilean Anti-neoliberal Uprising: A Catalyst for decolonial de-monumentalization. *Memory Studies, 14*(6), 1226–1240.

Bevins, V. (2023). *If We Burn: The Mass Protest Decade and the Missing Revolution*. Wildfire.

Caruth, C. (1996). *Unclaimed Experience. Trauma, Narrative, and History*. The Johns Hopkins University Press.

Copjec, J. (2015). *Read my Desire*. Verso.

Darrieussecq, M. (2023). *Sleepless*. Fitzcarraldo Editions.

De Vivanco, L., & Johansson, M. (Eds.). (2021). *Instantáneas en la Marcha*. Ediciones Universidad Alberto Hurtado.

Fernández, P. (2020). *Sobre la Marcha: Notas Acerca del Estallido Social en Chile*. Debate.

Freud, S. (2001a). Introductory lectures on psycho-analysis (1916–1917[1915–1917]). In *The Standard Edition of the Complete Psychological Works of Sigmund Freud, Vol. XV (1915–1916)*. Vintage.

Freud, S. (2001b). The interpretation of Dreams (second part). In *The Standard Edition of the Complete Psychological Works of Sigmund Freud, Vol. V (1900–1901)*. Vintage

Frosh, S. (2013). *Hauntings: Psychoanalysis and Ghostly Transmissions*. Palgrave Macmillan.

Grimmer, H. (2025). Reclaiming *el Pueblo*: The Role of Memories of the Unidad Popular in Artistic Interventions During the Chilean Revolt, 2019/20. In S. van den Elzen & A. Rigney (Eds.), *Memory and the Language of Contention*. Brill.

Lacan, J. (1997). *The Seminar of Jacques Lacan, Book III: The Psychoses, 1955–1956*. W. W. Norton & Company.

Lacan, J. (2017). *The Seminar of Jacques Lacan, Book V: Formations of the Unconscious*. Polity.

Lapping, C. (2011). *Psychoanalysis in Social Research*. Routledge.

Leader, D. (2019). *Why Can't We Sleep?* Penguin.
Llanos, B. (2021). Revuelta Social y Archivo Visual en el Chile Actual. *Contemporánea, 14*(1), 64–83.
López, M. (2021). Democracia e Igualdad Callejera: Acerca Del Octubre Chileno. In L. de Vivanco & M. Johansson (Eds.), *Instantáneas en la Marcha. Repertorio de las Movilizaciones en Chile.* Ediciones Universidad Alberto Hurtado.
Márquez, F. (2020). Por Una Antropología de los Escombros: El Estallido Social en Plaza Dignidad, Santiago de Chile. *Revista 180, 45*, 1–13.
McGowan, T. (2016). *Capitalism and Desire*. Columbia University Press.
Meruane, L. (2017). *Seeing Red*. Atlantic Books.
Meruane, L. (2021). *Zona Ciega.* Random House.
Müller, J.-W. (2024). On the square. *Philosophy & Social Criticism* (Online first).
Pinochet, C. (2021). Disrupting normalcy. Artistic Interventions and Political Mobilisation Against the Neoliberal City (Santiago, Chile, 2019). *Social Identities, 27*(5), 538–554.
Rose, J. (2004). *On Not Being Able to Sleep: Psychoanalysis and the Modern World*. Vintage.
San Martín, F., Macchiavello, C., & Solimano, P. (Eds.). (2023). *Dismantling the Nation: Contemporary Art in Chile.* Amherst College Press.
United Nations. (2019). *Report of the Mission to Chile 30 October - 22 November 2019.* Available at: https://www.ohchr.org/sites/default/files/Documents/Countries/CL/Report_Chile_2019_EN.pdf
Vanheule, S. (2011). A Lacanian Perspective on Psychotic Hallucinations. *Theory & Psychology, 21*(1), 86–106.
Žižek, S. (2023). *Too Late to Awaken. What Lies Ahead When There is no Future?* Allen Lane.

4

The Fantasy of Immediacy

This chapter continues my exploration of the libidinal economy of the *estallido* as it unfolds in the visual field. As I demonstrated in the previous chapter, seeing is often mistaken for a straightforward sensory process, yet it is in fact deeply entangled with the symbolic order. This entanglement means that our vision always involves the gaze of the Other—a source not of reassurance, but of unease and anxiety. Consequently, the visual field becomes a site where we can discern the imaginary narratives that allow the subject to locate its unconscious desire as a means of coping with the misrecognition emanating from the Other. My preceding interpretation of Nicolás' experience sheds light on how difficult it was to recognise oneself in the emancipatory wake-up call of the revolt. Although he consciously embraced the idea that 'Chile woke up', the associations elicited by the signifier 'dream' in his speech reveal an unconscious circuit of excess and antagonism underpinning his identification as an awakened subject. My material suggests, however, that the difficulties involved in responding to the call of the Other of the *estallido* can find more than one mode of expression in the visual field.

Police brutality and human rights violations formed the harrowing backdrop against which 'Chile woke up', as the previous

G. Sánchez, *A Rebel Unconscious*, Studies in the Psychosocial,
https://doi.org/10.1007/978-3-032-12275-9_4

chapter showed (Arensburg-Castelli et al., 2021). Several national and international organisations have contributed to contextualising the scale of state repression (INDH, 2019; Inter-American Commission on Human Rights, 2022). In the first two months of the popular uprising, over thirteen thousand people were admitted to accident and emergency departments with injuries sustained in the context of protest—three thousand of which were caused by firearms and other so-called less-lethal weapons. By 15 January 2020, 'the number of people with ocular trauma had reached 405, and 33 had suffered eye bursts, in some cases resulting in total loss of vision in both eyes' (Inter-American Commission on Human Rights, 2022, p. 62). For some researchers, the severity of the police response makes it difficult to treat it merely as a manoeuvre to restore public order (Landaeta & Herrero, 2021). The state clearly treated eyes as enemies, almost independently of the bodies to which they belonged. In this sense, it has been argued that the state sought to reassert control over the distribution of the visible by blinding protesters to what they had already seen: a mode of existence no longer in solidarity with neoliberalism (Durán & Vetö, 2021). Ironically, then, the excessive repression implicitly acknowledged that the experience of the end of neoliberalism was already materially underway.

The relationship between what was visible and what was not in the context of the revolt is at the centre of this chapter. Echoing the significance of information and communication technologies in other uprisings throughout the 2010s (Axford, 2011; Herrera, 2014; Mortensen, Neumayer & Poell, 2019), I focus on the unconscious dynamics elicited by the widespread reliance on social media during the *estallido*. Arguably, the most extended justification for the recording of videos and production of photographs was precisely to grant visibility to the excesses of state repression and to gather evidence that could eventually be used in court proceedings. This is something that traditional media did rather timidly, which earned them the distrust of the population. As a result, a partisan divide between 'them' and 'us' emerged. An example of this can be found in one of the few available books in English that address the aesthetics of the revolt. The authors quote the testimony of a protestor who claims that television and newspapers can no longer be trusted, insofar as they represent 'the state's agenda'. 'The agenda of the streets, the public's agenda', he clarifies, 'is written on the city's walls and on Instagram' (Gordon-Zolov & Zolov, 2022, p. 9). If, as María put it in the previous chapter, the walls were yelling at you on the street, then social media appears to exert a similar interpellative call. As my interpretation will show, the centrality of social media and digital platforms played an important role in the libidinal economy of the *estallido*.

My analysis pays attention to a singular aspect of the everyday experience of social media during the revolt. As Barrie Axford (2011) suggested in the context of the Arab Spring, the main aesthetic qualities of social media are immediacy and interactivity, features that were a source of both great potential and even greater scepticism. The latter stemmed largely from a sense of inauthenticity grounded in more traditional conceptions of political engagement—that is, a critique of social media's tendency to promote a form of politics perceived as detached from 'actual' events. Intriguingly, Axford's reflections point to something of a contradiction: the more social media allows protesters to experience immediacy, the more it simultaneously creates distance. It is fair to say that the scepticism surrounding the role of social media in the uprisings of the early 2010s had all but disappeared by 2019. During the *estallido*, the act of taking pictures and recording videos to share later on social media stopped being perceived as contravening the implicit manual of what a proper protester should be. Quite the opposite: as we shall see, it became an important way to recognise oneself within the shared experience of the end of neoliberalism. So much so, in fact, that at times it became difficult to determine where the recording device ended and the individual began:

> We took the streets over and raised our cell phones to warn them that we were listening to them, that we were their eyewitnesses, that we would be there vigilant so that nothing, nothing, NOTHING ever again, would go unregistered or be denied. Our cameras were eyes without eyelids or eyelashes cherishing evidence. (Meruane, 2021, p. 52)

What follows is an exploration of the fantasmatic supports underpinning the experience of merging oneself with cameras to the point of becoming eyes without eyelids. I proceed by taking up Anna Kornbluh's

(2024) argument that immediacy has come to define the dominant logic guiding the way we live. This means that different dimensions of our life—culture, politics, intimacy—have become increasingly regulated by an imperative to immersion grounded in the primacy of values such as intensity, instantaneity, and horizontality. According to Veronica Barassi (2015), in the context of protest, the immediacy of social media should be understood as an ambivalent temporalising practice: while it can operate as an important mechanism for organisation, it can also lead to severe curtailments of political effectiveness. This is why she urges us to study 'how people internalize the hegemonic temporality of immediacy and negotiate with it' (Barassi, 2015, p. 80). My argument below is that the ambivalence of immediacy can also be felt at a psychic level. When we take immediacy not as the reverse of mediation—as if we could simply shift from one to the other depending on the circumstances—but rather as the concealment of mediation, we open up the possibility for studying the psychic labour involved in removing the distance between our eyes and what we see.

Combating (Mis)Representation

A few days after the revolt began, the art gallery CIMA—'summit' in English—launched a significant project that catapulted it into the limelight. Taking advantage of its location at the top of a building directly abutting Dignity Square, the gallery installed a camera that recorded the activity around the square uninterruptedly and broadcast the live footage via its YouTube channel. The camera was christened 'CENTINELA'—'sentinel' or 'sentry'—a term derived from the French *sentinelle*, first used in the late 1500s to describe someone keeping guard or a military watchtower defending a city. A sentinel is a watchman, often a soldier, whose remit is to monitor the position entrusted to her or him—in short, someone for whom no action can go unseen. CENTINELA's motto was: 'to observe, communicate, and persist is an act of resistance'. The logic underpinning this project is briefly described on its YouTube channel: the camera's aim is to 'show live the reality of the demonstrations' for an audience 'interested in the truth that the hegemonic press doesn't show', thus creating 'a historical archive born out of urgency, ensuring the permanence of memory within everyone's reach'. CIMA's project can be understood, then, as a manoeuvre to counter the dissemination of the state's agenda through the hegemonic media by directly and continuously broadcasting the revolt.

Settling the debate about when the *estallido* ended is presumably an infructuous endeavour. The waning of its energy at the beginning of 2020 is irrefutable, and the severe limitations on social interaction imposed by the political response to the pandemic marked, for many, a point of no return. Yet this is far from a consensus. There are, however, certain milestones to consider. In September 2022, the Chilean people categorically rejected the draft of a new constitution written by a democratically elected committee with a majority of left-wing members. The 'world's most progressive constitution', as the headline of an article in The Guardian put it,[1] went straight into the bin—along with much of the transformational spirit of the revolt. CENTINELA, nonetheless, continued to record. The fact that no demonstrator had set foot on the square in the months preceding the referendum did not appear to be a strong enough reason to stop. Indeed, the recording carried on uninterruptedly for at least another two years. CIMAS's project, this sort of officially unofficial broadcaster of the revolt, exhibited an unwavering commitment to its goal that is worth exploring further.

The continuous recording of a revolt that had already ceased cannot be attributed to an oversight on the part of the sentinel. In December 2021, the members of CIMA took part in an online conversation about CENTINELA.[2] Among the many interesting details of their work, they mentioned that the idea of livestreaming the square day and night emerged spontaneously once they finally gained access to the building, a few days after the uprising had begun. They tried several cameras but ended up damaging their batteries as none of them were designed to record nonstop. Once they found the right one, they immediately recognised how important it was to have an 'objective image' independent of the vested interests of traditional media. Furthermore, a growing sense

[1] https://www.theguardian.com/world/2022/sep/04/constitution-approve-vote-chile.

[2] https://www.youtube.com/watch?v=ldZGjc79394.

of responsibility emerged among them with the realisation that many people were vicariously experiencing the revolt through their recordings. This is why they did not stop. As Trinidad Lopetegui said during the conversation: 'At no point we questioned if we should stop. It was more about navigating emotions [...], because the mission and the commitment was so big'. Making the revolt immediately visible developed into a responsibility—much like a sentry enjoined to stand guard to the point of becoming indistinguishable from their post.

In the most intense months of the *estallido*, CIMA's project stood as the pinnacle of efforts to counterbalance the revolt's representation on mainstream platforms. 'There's no decent mass media in this country', said Rodrigo, a senior academic. His stance was a common one among the people I interviewed. As soon as the words left his mouth, he recoiled from the moralising undertones of his statement and qualified it by adding that the media simply 'aren't up to the task'. It is worth emphasising that this is not merely a disagreement over the angle from which events were presented; the task Rodrigo refers to is the silence surrounding human rights violations. Accompanied by a telling and apparently unintended pun, Isabel—who appeared in the previous chapter—offered a description of the situation: 'Twitter exploded, I mean, Twitter was the way to find out what was happening, you know? The issue of human rights violations would have been impossible to know without Twitter because there was no other way'. The *estallido*, so to speak, detonated twice; insofar as the explosion on the streets was not being properly recorded, a virtual explosion occurred on social media.

Let us look more closely at this duality. Arturo is a PhD researcher interested in the unfolding of visual memory in the revolt. At several points during our interviews, he emphasises that 'the *estallido* is mainly a visual thing; it's an extremely visual phenomenon'. For him, this feature is contingent on the contemporary importance attributed to social media. Like most of my interviewees, he links this characteristic to the cleavage between state and people: 'There's the official discourse, propagated by the news, the newspapers, for example, that presents an image of the *estallido*, but we have these other images that circulate on social media; the videos, the pictures, the selfies'. The frontier separating 'them' from 'us' is thus a dispute over the visualisation of the revolt, the manner in which the latter is translated into images. This position can be perceived as a reversal of the activity at the base of the fantasy of sleeplessness: whereas that position aims to forbear from defining the revolt by refusing its translation into a stable image, here the goal is to incessantly capture the event in order to reveal the truth obfuscated by the misleading mediation of the official discourse.

Recourse to the oppositions between state/people or official/alternative as a way of justifying the impulse to record and broadcast the revolt can also be found in other parallel events (Bevins, 2023). The uprisings in Tunisia in 2010, Egypt in 2011, and Lebanon in 2019—the latter occurring literally the day before the Chilean *estallido*—exhibit a strikingly similar pattern, despite the significant differences in the oppressiveness of their respective governments compared to Chile (El-Fattah, 2021; Herrera, 2014; Kozman, 2023). In all these cases, social media played a role in organising demonstrations, disseminating information, and denouncing police brutality and human rights violations. Arturo's account follows this same logic: 'That's why the use of pictures and videos was so important during the revolt: many allegations, for example, were made thanks to pictures and videos'. This is, without a shadow of a doubt, an accurate description of how things unfolded during the *estallido*. From day one, I myself recall dreading picking up my phone in the morning because I already knew what awaited me: dozens of videos showing unmerciful and remorseless police officers engaged in what can only be described as carnage. Yet, as disheartening as this was, it was important to know. This is why, for Arturo, 'the use of the camera in the *estallido* was very important'.

His speech, however, also allows us to glimpse other effects derived from this dynamic. Since he moved from the idea of vision to that of a recording device, I asked him, following the last quotation, to develop that train of thought further. His answer was the following:

> Yeah, cos, above all [*todo*] the camera on your phone, I mean, the fact that we now have a camera on our phone and we can record everything [*todo*] at all [*todo*] times, and all [*todos*] of us, I believe, have recordings of being on the streets, or we have collected pictures, let's say, of what the demonstrations were like.

The foregoing may seem like an unremarkable vignette. Indeed, it appears to be a rather uninspired description of what most Chileans involved in demonstrations must have done, and so at first glance, it does not seem worth pondering in much detail. Yet the fashion in which this generalised activity is conveyed hints at significant symbolic associations. In the confined space of just two lines, Arturo's speech becomes saturated with a single signifier: '*todo*', a word that can mean 'all', 'everything', or 'whole'. Since we now carry a camera with us 'everywhere' we go, we can record 'everything' we see, a practice that, today, 'everybody' engages in. In practical terms, we are identical to the camera, a device that sees everything and, by extension, so should we. Even the first iteration of *todo*, intended as a simple emphatic connector—'above all [*todo*] the camera on your mobile…'—is illustrative. Taken literally, does this not echo CIMA's project? Just like the sentinel's lens hovering over 'everyone' in Dignity Square, Arturo's camera is also positioned above 'everything'.

The Duty of Seeing Everything

This unanticipated and cramped eruption of the signifier of totality is far from anecdotal. Carmen is another doctoral researcher I interviewed. She will make an important appearance in Chapter 6, so I will spare some details here. The revolt found her in Europe, where she had just begun her master's degree at a prestigious university and, after an initial period of hesitation, she resolved to study the *estallido* as the topic of her dissertation. As she revisited that period during our interview, she described an abrupt mood swing. At first, before engaging with the uprising as a research subject, she deliberately kept herself away from the news. 'For my own mental health', she acknowledged, 'my decision was to stop looking at Instagram, stop looking at Twitter, to take some distance and focus on my experience there'. Not seeing became her strategy for remaining mentally in one piece—a completely reasonable and deeply relatable choice. She then opted to study the *estallido* and things moved quickly from there. That decision, she said, 'meant an important change because I kinda threw myself into receiving all [*toda*] the information that I had originally closed myself off to'. At this very point, a memory surfaced—her decision to study the revolt coincided with her starting to jog. So she goes:

> I started jogging, to enlarge the cliché even more (laughs), and, and I jogged while listening to podcasts, podcasts, podcasts, podcasts about everything [*todo*], and all [*todo*] this to understand what the fuck was happening in this country. But also endless calls with friends, so they could tell me how was… like everything [*todo*], everything [*todo*]; I was trying to connect more with how things were lived here, and discuss all [*todo*] about politics with everyone [*todos*], in every [*todo*] possible way. It was like opening up again and I started reading a lot, even if little had been produced – I mean, cos there was not much academic production at that point – but like all [*todas*] kinds of experiences – everything [*todo*], everything [*todo*] served me for that purpose.

After her initial refusal to see, deciding to study the revolt made her want to see everything. But not just that. When we place Arturo's line about mobile phones ('… we can record everything [*todo*] at all [*todo*] times, and all [*todos*] of us, I believe, have recordings') alongside Carmen's passage about chatting with friends ('… and discuss all [*todo*] about politics with everyone [*todos*], in every [*todo*] possible way') a staggering structural equivalence becomes apparent. Here, seeing everything is not enough. Both converge on the idea that everything must be seen all the time and from every angle. Meruane's triple 'nothing' quoted in the first section of this chapter ('nothing, nothing, NOTHING ever again, would go unregistered'), finds in the experiences of Arturo and Carmen an almost direct, positive correlation—since *every* front is covered at *all* times, *everything* becomes visible.

One aspect of Carmen's excerpt seems worth further emphasis. Her recollection begins with an activity ostensibly unrelated to the rest of the narrative: jogging. She refers to this in strictly colloquial terms; she was enjoying herself in a new city and, at some point, took advantage of the city's amenities to start exercising. Significantly, her eagerness to engage in physical activity emerged precisely at the moment she resolved to research the revolt. Moreover, from the range of options available to her, she chose to run. All of this may, of course, be a fortuitous coincidence, yet there is enough room to rehearse an alternative reading. When our eyes scan the ten reiterations of '*todo*' in the transcribed vignette, do we not get the impression that she is, in effect, running on a symbolic plane? The seemingly endless repetition of the same word, line after line, evokes a pursuit—the ceaseless attempt to reach the next iteration as quickly as possible. For Carmen, seeing everything from every angle at all times places her on a sort of symbolic treadmill, permanently accelerating so as not to lose sight of the next 'everything'.

As tempting as it might be to draw parallels between this insatiable appetite for seeing everything and the figure of the panopticon, a crucial difference must be noted. As is well known, Michel Foucault posited the panopticon as the linchpin of disciplinary society. He identified in Bentham's architectural project of surveillance the dissociation of the see/being seen dyad: in this prison, the inmate is seen but does not see that they are being seen. For Foucault, panoptic spatial arrangements are laboratories of power insofar as they allow an infinitesimal distribution of power relations. The separation of the see/being seen dyad, therefore, means that even if surveillance is discontinuous, its effects are nonetheless permanent. The reason for this is simple: surveillance has been internalised. Accordingly, Foucault (1995, p. 201) claims that 'inmates should be caught up in a power situation of which they are themselves the bearers'. Like the panopticon, the impetus for an uninterrupted recording of the revolt also aspires to achieve full visibility—in this case, against the partiality of the official view. Unlike the panopticon, however, this process is not sustained by the division inherent in the see/being seen dyad. If something is internalised here, it is not the fear of being seen, *but the desire for the Other to see me as someone who sees everything*. Consequently, recording the revolt implies being seen seeing—a particular mix of exhibitionism and voyeurism.

The final example that helps me fully delineate this dynamic comes from another PhD researcher: Daniela. She is a historian, a leftist militant, and someone not particularly lucky, considering that the month before the revolt began she injured her knee. As a result, she had to devise intricate strategies in order to partake in demonstrations, as she never hesitated about being part of them. The crutches she needed to get around posed a significant obstacle not only to completing the rally's route, but even more so to a quick getaway in case the situation on the street got out of hand—which was more the rule than the exception. Despite her precautionary measures, several times she found herself in unsafe surroundings. Yet her commitment never wavered.

In our interviews, she devoted a good amount of time to talking about her own experience and that of her friends on the streets—all the while consistently highlighting the importance of images in shaping that experience. In a line tantamount to Arturo's, she remarked that the revolt 'was totally a visual event, I think, and social media as well and the use of the internet and all that spread it like, booom! tremendously'. She then compared this situation with the dictatorship, referring to the 2006 documentary *The City of Photographers*, which revolves around the significance of a group of lensmen in recording various facets of totalitarian oppression on the streets. For her, the circumstances are dramatically different inasmuch as, in 2019, 'everybody is a photographer', so 'now we could all do something and doing it was a duty [*deber*]'. I asked her to expand on this precise idea. For the sake of readability, my interpretation will proceed by dividing her full answer into two vignettes.

> *How come [a duty]?*
> Like, to record it, you know? Like the recording becomes… recording as a duty [*deber*], as if you see [*ves*] someone being beaten up you had to record it, and in many cases, for the accusation, people were like: "Does anyone have photos of this or that moment?" Like the accusation that could later be made through the National Institute of Human Rights had to – for the most part, though not necessarily, but hopefully – have a recording of what happened because that gave it more validity. And since everyone [*todos*] has recordings of everything [*todo*], we looked out for them: "Hey, in such and such corner", whatever. For example, what happened to this guy who fell into a hole in downtown Santiago, which is terrible because one of my dear friends was running alongside him and saw when he fell, and she was running next to the guy, you know? And she was running and suddenly poof! the guy disappeared, mate. And she told me that she kept on running, you know? She kept on running, and the bloke died. And she told me: "Fuck! If I only had had like the recording of that". Like if she had been running and recording the thing – which is kinda crazy, but there are people who do it (laughs).

The excerpt confronts us, yet again, with the same rationale behind the act of recording discernible in the accounts of Arturo and Carmen, that is, fighting back against police brutality and the official (mis)construction of the revolt's visual landscape. Moreover, Daniela reiterates the association I have been stressing in my interpretation: everyone recording everything. Her reply, however, introduces other crucial associations. My intervention for further clarification was prompted by the sudden appearance of the signifier 'duty', which entered the conversation seemingly out of the blue. Subsequently, she insisted on the equivalence recording = duty, a formulation that aligns with the figure of the sentinel resisting the government's oppression—when they are blinding demonstrators, you ought to do something. But when we isolate this signifier from the discourse formation that provides its imaginary stabilisation, other interpretive possibilities begin to emerge.

Daniela deploys the term '*deber*', a polysemic notion. As mentioned above, her clear intention is to convey a strong sense of duty—a collective responsibility for combating the state's repression through multimedia recordings. Unlike in English though, *deber* in Spanish also means 'being indebted'. A case can be made, then, that this kind of accountability for the other in the revolt (*deber* as duty) comes with a perception of liability (*deber* as indebtedness); something is owed or due. But with a small twist, even a third association appears. Through a scansion, *deber* can be turned into *de-ver*, two words phonetically indistinguishable from the former that mean 'to see'. Taking into account these three possibilities, a significant displacement becomes noticeable. By approaching 'everything' not as an indefinite pronoun referring to a total number of things, but rather as a signifier with autonomous existence in the symbolic, we are in position to uncover an unconscious aspect of this ceaseless recording. In order to recognise themselves in the call of the revolt, these subjects made of seeing an act that was *immediately* recording. Recording was a duty (*deber*) because, within the experience of the end of neoliberalism, recording was already 'to see' (*de-ver*)—and failing to do so renders us indebted (*deber*).

The imaginary homologation of seeing and recording is what I refer to as *the fantasy of immediacy*. It functions as an imaginary way of resolving the mystery of what the Other of the *estallido* wants from us. Within this framework, vision becomes libidinised by being made into a site of plenitude. This does not mean that people were pleased with what they had to see, but that seeing was the right thing to do—and that is why they had to see in the same way that a camera is capable of recording everything. At this point, we can perceive how this 'everything' differs from the discursive formation in which seeing everything means that the more recordings we gather, the greater the chances are of holding the police accountable for their misconduct. In a material sense, 'everything' serves as the currency of what is owed—something we must accumulate in order to pay it back. This might explain why running tends to accompany narrations of 'everything'. The fact that subjects were chasing and collecting 'everything' in a symbolic sense becomes tragically clear in the anecdote of Daniela's friend—an association made by someone who, due to her knee injury, could not run during the revolt. On 27 December 2019, a 33-year-old construction worker who was escaping from the police's deterrence tactics fell into a power line pit filled with water and died. Daniela's friend was running next to him. At a moment in which she could have imagined literally anything—imagine, for instance, him not falling into the pit—she bemoaned not having a recording of the tragedy. Not recording amounts to the unimaginable. So, at least unconsciously, all she could do was carry on running, in search of the next 'everything'.

This libidinal investment in the recording finds its final confirmation in Daniela's justification of the duty of seeing. She illustrates the weight of responsibility involved in documenting the revolt by referring to the complaints submitted through the National Institute of Human Rights. As mentioned at the beginning of this chapter, organisations like this played a key role in putting the state repression into perspective. Nonetheless, the initial peremptory nature of this injunction is drastically qualified in the same line: visual evidence was mandatory 'for the most part, though not necessarily, but hopefully', since that would give it 'more validity'. Regardless of how accurate this assessment may be, an internal inconsistency surfaces in her speech through her dithering—a vacillation that signals a dimension of this duty that extends beyond its consciously acknowledged justifications. In a way, recording everything was excessive not only because police brutality reached new heights during the *estallido*, but also because many developed an excessive relationship with sight as a means of locating themselves within the revolt.

Replying to the Other's Impossible Call

Daniela's reply, as I mentioned, was a long and significant one. Another example came to her mind as soon as she finished talking about her friend. Without a pause, she proceeded to share the experience of her partner's flatmates, who worked in the production industry and devoted time and energy to recording the revolt. Her associations are, once again, immensely rich.

> And the other thing is that just at that time, I was in close contact with some guys, and one of them began to record daily videos of the *estallido*. I have the Instagram and everything [*todo*] if you want it later; they are remarkable. So, I saw how he came home, where I stayed – my partner lived with him – and then said: "Alright, I'm gonna start editing", and bum! He edited and made some beautiful videos, you know?, with everything [*todo*] that had happened that day. He put in, like, an intro; it was like the kind of thing like when you go to an event, an event like about whatever, like ermmm, like an event like, I think, I don't know… I'm gonna go to the CLACSO [conference, in Mexico], then you're gonna go to this thing and the first day a video will come out, like a recording – it's like a ritual recording. Of course, it has a logic of recording it, but it is also like a ritual you're in. But at some point, it turned weird; you've been making videos for 15 days, this guy was like, of course, "Nah, I can't do it every [*todos*] day", that is, "I can't anymore, I can't go to the rallies every [*todos*] day either". Suddenly, man, "I've been going for 15 days, 20 days, I'm tired, I'm gonna stay here". That was strange, like missing one day.

My attention is drawn to two aspects of this quotation: the deployment of the terms 'event' and 'ritual'. Daniela received first-hand knowledge about the crafting of videos on the *estallido*—these beautiful videos containing everything [*todo*] that happened on the street. At the moment she begins to describe the editing process, her words all of a sudden seem to vanish. She refers to the revolt as an 'event' but as soon as she makes that association, she evidently struggles to continue ('an event like about whatever, like ermmm, like an event like, I think, I don't know'); almost as if mediation via editing could not be part of the narration. Something does come to her mind though. Daniela makes a symbolic bridge between this event and an academic one: the Latin American Council of Social Sciences (CLACSO) conference, which she would attend later that year. Established in 1967, CLACSO encompasses almost 1,000 postgraduate and research centres in 56 countries. Among its explicit aims, the promotion, development, and consolidation of critical thinking are paramount. Its annual conference, the one Daniela alludes to, is the region's biggest hub of radical academic knowledge. And yet, all this is reduced in her speech to a clip, a 'ritual recording'.

The revolt can indeed be described as an event, that is, as the opening up of a new and unforeseeable horizon of possibilities. However, in Daniela's speech, the *estallido* is not granted such a lofty status. Quite the contrary, her use of 'event' is closer to that of a social occasion, an event planning—much like a well-organised academic conference. This latter sense of 'event' emerges, it is important to highlight, when the revolt is turned into a video. 'Everything' is meticulously edited, framed within a certain narrative, synchronised with the music; it is transformed into a spellbinding offering to the eyes. However, and apparently in the same way we do with academic conferences, it becomes ritualised. Daniela draws two equivalences here: revolt = conference = event, on the one hand, and revolt = conference = ritual, on the other. The link between them is the act of recording. And at this precise point, we can detect a tone of disappointment in her response. She begins with an animated description of the recordings, only to see such enthusiasm dissolve into convention. A ritual is precisely that: a set of rules organising a ceremony. Rituals are solemn acts people have become accustomed to; nothing within a ritual is out of the ordinary, as the rules are explicitly in place to prevent such an outcome. In an ironic twist, the *estallido*—that transformative event if ever there was one in Chile—was discursively turned into a custom for the sake of its own preservation.

The last part of the vignette can be understood as the combined subjective effect of the three *deber*: the duty, the act of seeing, and indebtedness. Daniela reaches the end of her reply sounding dejected. Something seemed off to her; after a certain number of videos, her friends can no longer keep up with 'everything', and tiredness set in. 'That was strange, like missing one day' is how the quotation ends. I asked her what she felt in that situation, and she was emphatic: 'Guilt, you feel guilty'. Here, she shifts to her experience, and the feeling of being in debt protrudes: 'I've got things to do, you know? I can't be on the street every [*todo*] day; there was a point when it was like, like it was no longer possible'. Daniela's account differs very little from what someone behind on their payments might say, the only discrepancy is the nature of the fee. From the particular angle adopted in my interpretation, the revolt's currency is 'everything'. Based on the experiences analysed above, the virtually interminable succession of images, videos, and selfies around the *estallido* was, among other things, a way of responding to a call of duty. Answering this call involved an unconscious attachment: the libidinal investment in our sight as that which would make us *immediately* coincide with what the Other wants from us.

My interpretation suggests that what supports this dynamic is the fantasy of immediacy. In each of the experiences explored above, the sublimation of recording 'everything' as one of the most important activities during the revolt is discernible. This is presented as an act of resistance—and, at a conscious level, it definitely was. Nonetheless, the imaginary kernel of this process is that, irrespective of the accuracy of the claim, a crucial aspect is selectively obfuscated: mediation. The divide they/us sustaining the rationalisations of the permanent recordings maintains that the *estallido* has been wrongly or partially represented by a media apparatus subservient to the state's agenda. In opposition, millions of recording devices on the street attempted to present (not re-present) the revolt in itself. Somehow, despite all their crafting, engineering, broadcasting, and editing, let alone the fact that a device stands between us and what we see, these recordings are perceived as direct and unmediated expressions of the revolt. To the state/people and official/alternative cleavages that organise the discourses around the recording of the event, we must append the imaginary mediated/unmediated frontier.

By following and isolating some of the terms used by my interviewees to narrate their experiences, we can access a different libidinal economy underpinning the visual reality of the revolt—one distinct from the fantasy of sleeplessness. As I have insisted, recording everything on the street was not merely an activity but also a signifier, that is, a symbolic piece allowing subjects to navigate the desire of the Other of the *estallido.* They felt interpellated as subjects who have the duty [*deber*] to see [*de-ver*] everything [*todo*], an experience made possible by phones, which imaginarily homologate seeing and recording. So, unlike Nicolás and the fantasy of sleeplessness, Arturo, Carmen, and Daniela *did try* to respond to this interpellation, which nonetheless proved excessive. In other words, faced with the desiring call of the Other of the *estallido*, they sought to solve the mystery of this call by identifying with the duty of seeing, while elevating 'everything' to a different symbolic dignity—an unconscious mechanism to regain recognition amid the experience of the end of neoliberalism. Within this fantasmatic realm, where 'everything' is the currency used to pay our symbolic debt, they squared an impasse with their conscious life by reproducing an original impossibility. They became the bearers of something that should not be there: the mediators of immediacy.

The fantasy of immediacy is the problematic solution to the belief that mediation is exclusively a property of power structures. In a word, mediation is invariably deceitful. Since that is the case, the incessant recording of the revolt can be interpreted as an unconscious attempt to turn representation into the direct presentation of facts. This is why the uninterrupted nature of this endeavour is crucial—everything must be recorded from every corner, *at all times*. The ceaselessness of mediation is what ultimately sustains the illusion of immediacy. But, at the same time, it gives birth to a hoarder subject for whom the accumulation of recordings becomes the ultimate goal. The cases of Arturo, Carmen, and Daniela analysed here hint at a kind of rapacious disposition to have it all, an acquisitive propensity for stockpiling 'everything'. However, their own experiences indicate that this is an impossible enterprise. The sustenance of the imaginary of immediacy requires an indefatigable subject who, needless to say, does not exist.

In order to maintain the imaginary frontier of immediacy, within this libidinally charged narrative, truth is equated with the factual—although a very ad hoc notion of the latter. Unintentionally, the revolt becomes a sort of pristine phenomenon that must remain untouched, immaculate. Through this feature of the fantasy of immediacy, we can understand how the visual manufacturing of the *estallido*—under the guise of a call of duty—is subjectively perceived as non-mediated. Lina Meruane neatly captures this rejection of mediation through the idea of becoming 'eyes without eyelids or eyelashes cherishing evidence'. It is as though, in order to resist, we should face no resistance whatsoever. In the end, what the fantasy of immediacy fails to recognise is the noncoincidence between factual and truth. When mediation becomes synonymous with power, as is the case here, a fetishisation of facts takes shape—protestors resolve into de facto empiricists. As I have shown, this is a fantasmatic scenario insofar as the only way of dodging symbolic mediation is, so to speak, by turning a blind eye to it. Returning to the beginning of this section, CIMA's project eloquently epitomises the fantasy of immediacy. The sentinel was the subjective prototype springing from this fantasy, yet only a machine could do the job. And, since the camera cannot feel the pang of guilt of indebtedness, that eye without eyelids or eyelashes, freed from any restriction, continued patrolling the roundabout. It carried on seeing everything, even if 'everything' was no longer there.

Resisting Resistance

The interpretation I have offered in this chapter continues my exploration of the idea that there was no 'brute vision' during the uprising and, consequently, that seeing was not a straightforward activity. This is the case not only because we are always exposed to contingent and asymmetrical distributions of the visible and the invisible, but also, and crucially, because human beings do not look with their eyes but with their desire. The visual field, simply put, is as incomplete as the discursive field. So, just as we require imaginary supplements to stabilise meaning, seeing stands in need of a fantasmatic formation for its support. By treating certain speech units—particularly 'everything' and 'duty'—as signifiers that can move autonomously and develop associations beyond the conscious intention of the speaker, I have reconstructed the fantasy of immediacy. In the wake of the experience of the end of neoliberalism, this imaginary narrative allowed subjects to secure recognition by directly turning vision into a site of resistance. This manoeuvre sought to consciously fight back against police brutality and the informational bias of traditional media—arguably the most conspicuous expressions of external opposition to the rebelliousness of protesters. And yet, it cannot be said that this was the clash of two fully positive forces or positions. 'Everything' is the material leftover of this attempt at becoming one with our position in the form of eyes without eyelashes—it is what psychically resists resistance, so to speak. This is the manifestation of the rebelliousness of the unconscious.

The above should make us cautious about assuming that the interpretation of visual phenomena can be exhausted by power-centred models. A brief theoretical detour is needed here. One of the clearest expositions of how power relates to the visual comes from Gilles Deleuze's seminar on Foucault. According to Deleuze (2018), Foucault's project can be regarded as a philosophical approach to history, in the sense that he tried to distil the conditions of possibility for historical behaviours and mentalities to exist in the first place. These conditions are visibility and enunciability—what can be seen and what can be said. These are heterogeneous conditions that nonetheless presuppose each other. For Deleuze, a historical formation can be understood as the particular way in which visibility and enunciability are articulated; different combinations of what can be seen and said shape the coherence of our experience in the world. This is what Foucault calls 'knowledge', namely, the mutual capture between these heterogeneous conditions that renders both vision and discourse meaningful. If we can say that something is 'true', it is because there is a correspondence between what can be said and seen, on one side, and a historical knowledge formation, on the other.

From this perspective, knowledge is not something an individual possesses but the very condition of our historical experience. Deleuze (2018, p. 41) is categorical on this point: 'there is nothing underneath knowledge or before knowledge'. There is no experience that is not already a combination of ways of seeing and saying. For a regime of knowledge to be imposed, there must be a power capable of making things visible and sayable. Power, therefore, does not have a form in itself, but it can produce a formation by rendering things visible and sayable in a particular manner. Consequently: 'Everything that is done in an era can only be done if it comes to light' (p. 26). We can see and say everything that a historical formation grants visibility and sayability to. Deleuze is strict about the disjunction between seeing and saying—so much so that, for him, it is of little interest to describe what one sees, unless one is speaking to someone who is blind. 'Because', he argues, 'if it is someone who sees the same thing as you, it does not seem very interesting to say what you see: "Wow! A ship", right?' (p. 29). All we can see is already visible.

Following Deleuze, politics is a matter of challenging the current regime of power-knowledge as a way to see and speak otherwise. The experience of the end of neoliberalism appears to fit this definition neatly. Chile woke up and we started to see and speak differently. Words like 'dignity', 'evasion', 'first line', and 'waking up' acquired entirely new meanings, while we simultaneously felt as though we were seeing everything with new eyes. Nevertheless, based on my interpretation, it is worth questioning whether talking about what one sees truly lacks interest, as Deleuze staunchly maintains. The point is not merely that two people standing in front of a ship may differ in what they see, but that—even if they both see the same ship—the word 'ship' has a materiality beyond the speaker's conscious control. The associations that 'ship' may carry are related to the historical formation we inhabit, but are not reducible to it. My interpretation clearly demonstrates this. The more the people I interviewed tried to show me how futile it was so say 'Wow! A ship'—because they obviously saw it—the more 'ship' acquired an autonomy that revealed that the experience of the revolt was not a confrontation between two positive or fully realised forms of visibility.

What Deleuze's approach to knowledge fails to acknowledge is the recognition of recognition, that is to say, the role of the Other. Visibility is all there is because identification, in terms of seeing and saying, cannot fail; hence the obviousness of the ship. From this perspective, to say that we wanted to see everything during the revolt is indeed an inconsequential statement, because everything is all we can ever see. In contrast, if we accept that the visual field is linked to the symbolic, then wanting to see 'everything' becomes crucial to the study of how recognition was secured in the scopic experience of the *estallido*. Fundamentally, for power-centred models like the one defended by Deleuze, there is nothing to secure since we are always dealing with fulfilled or actualised positions that will eventually meet resistance from another fulfilled or actualised position. All there is, is to win or lose. The psychic labour involved in the fantasy of immediacy, in contrast, suggests that this is not quite the case. There is something that resists resistance, and it can be grasped in the uncooperative disposition of certain words—we say 'Wow! A ship', and by the time we attempt to exert control over our words, that ship has sailed.

With the above in mind, let me return to the fantasy of immediacy. At first glance, at the level of meaning, it appears as the antipode to the fantasy of sleeplessness. Rather than a sheer reluctance to capture the revolt in images, the goal here is to record it continuously. In this sense, CIMA's counter-hegemonic project CENTINELA stands as the realisation of the motto 'Chile woke up': the possibility of eyes that never sleep. Explicitly presented as an attempt to break with the misinformation propagated by traditional media regarding human rights violations, its aim was to expose the divide between the state's agenda and that of the people. Put differently, this can be understood as a collective endeavour to resist state surveillance through a generalised sousveillance—the practice of watching 'from below', a kind of inverted surveillance in which the surveillors themselves become the watched (Fernback, 2013). Subjectively, however, this act of resistance entailed sinuous unconscious dynamics. As the experiences of Arturo, Carmen, and Daniela show, confronting the power of the state transformed the act of seeing into an unrelenting duty—one that plunged people into a permanent state of symbolic indebtedness.

What is fundamentally at stake in the fantasy of immediacy is the relationship between visibility and knowledge in its conventional sense. Since traditional media is deliberately not showing—i.e., making invisible—significant aspects of what is happening on the streets, part of the population remains ignorant of human rights violations and police brutality. The lack of knowledge identified in this narrative is remedied not simply through visibility, but through *permanent* visibility. This sort of checkmate move against institutional power rests on a problematic assumption: that the revolt has been so selective and tendentiously represented that we are left with no option but to embark on its direct presentation. This relentless recording without intermediaries—epitomised by CIMA's project—is cast as the means of revealing the truth that hegemonic media conceals. Therefore, truth comes to mean (a) something always visible, and (b) something always unmediated, so that mediation and invisibility are rendered synonymous with power strategies. However, the more the subject feels compelled to see everything, the heavier the psychic burden of erasing its own mediation becomes.

The fantasy of immediacy exhibits the psychic toll of conflating ideology with mediation and facts with truth. Guided by the assumption that mediation is invariably an ideological manoeuvre that ensnares the subject in power relations, the imperative to see everything culminates in a subjective impasse. The root of this impasse can be found in the semiotic structure of the visual field. While the idea that representation is deceptive holds a certain validity, this is not because something lies behind the veil of ideology that can be accessed directly or immediately. As Copjec (2015) reminds us, nothing stands behind representation, *and yet* it always seems to conceal something on account of the deceptiveness of language itself. Misrecognition is then unavoidable in the visual field, and what we cannot see is the way our desire distorts what we see. This is the opacity—the stain, in Lacanian jargon—that the fantasy of immediacy attempts to abolish: the effort to erase the gaze of the revolt. This fantasy conflates the eye with the gaze, refusing to acknowledge that seeing is inherently unsatisfying. As Lacan (1998, p. 103) asserts, '*you never look at me from the place from which I see you*' and, simultaneously, '*what I look at is never what I wish to see*'. The sensation of being trapped on a treadmill, endlessly chasing the infinite instantiations of 'everything', attests to the inescapability of desire in the visual field—'everything' is the symbolic obstacle to any immediate coincidence with our position, precisely the materiality that resists being recorded, no matter how hard we try.

The fantasy of immediacy offers a desiring narrative that stands in opposition to the fantasy of sleeplessness. This contrast becomes evident when we consider both as ways of confronting what Caruth (1996) describes to as the trauma of awakening—the simultaneous necessity and impossibility of responding to someone's call. On one hand, the fantasy of sleeplessness accepts this impossibility (I can never find recognition in the Other's call) but not its necessity (I nonetheless must wake up). On the other hand, the fantasy of immediacy acknowledges its necessity (I must wake up) but refuses its impossibility (I never wake up at the right time). The fantasy of sleeplessness begins with the acceptance that misrecognition is unavoidable. Unable to respond appropriately to the interpellation of the Other of the *estallido*, the subject unconsciously identifies with the caller rather than with the call itself. The libidinisation of the dream functions as a way of 'solving' the dilemma that answering the interpellation is not optional. By contrast, within the imaginary formation of the fantasy of immediacy, the subject goes to great unconscious lengths to *fully recognise itself* in the call of the Other. The libidinisation of the act of recording to see 'everything' is an attempt to become a constantly awakened subject, a process that must refuse any misrecognition.

As my interpretation evinces, despite their apparent opposition—avoiding any image in one case, and permanent recording in the other—both imaginary formations spring from the difficulties to deal with the emancipatory call of the Other of the *estallido*. They organise libidinal economies that allow the subject to cope with this process. For these subjects who have self-bound themselves to the good of a post-neoliberal society and shape themselves accordingly, the desire for social change seems admissible only in an unalloyed form. Either we reject it to the extent that we know it cannot be as pure as we wish (fantasy of sleeplessness), or we accept it only insofar as it is direct and unmediated (fantasy of immediacy). Yet these remain problematic solutions, since they first must accept what they ultimately reject; it is through this partial acceptance and partial rejection that these subjects manage to imaginarily frame their desire for social change.

References

Arensburg-Castelli, S., Barrientos-Delgado, J., Astudillo-Lizama, P., & Venegas, D. (2021). Police Violence: Sexual Political Dehumanisation Strategies used by Chilean Gendered Institutions. *Social Identities, 27*(5), 593–607.

Axford, B. (2011). Talk About a Revolution: Social Media and the MENA Uprisings. *Globalizations, 8*(5), 681–686.

Barassi, V. (2015). Social Media, Immediacy and the Time for Democracy: Critical Reflections on Social Media as 'Temporalizing Practices'. In L. Dencik & O. Leistert (Eds.), *Critical Perspectives on Social Media and Protest: Between Control and Emancipation.* Rowman & Littlefield International.

Bevins, V. (2023). *If We Burn: The Mass Protest Decade and the Missing Revolution.* Wildfire.

Caruth, C. (1996). *Unclaimed Experience. Trauma, Narrative, and History.* The Johns Hopkins University Press.

Copjec, J. (2015). *Read my Desire*. Verso.

Deleuze, G. (2018). *El Saber. Curso Sobre Foucault, Tomo 1.* Editorial Cactus.

Durán, C., & Vetö, S. (2021). La 'Rostridad' en el estallido Social Chileno de 2019: Acerca de la Estrategia Político-Policial de Mutilación Ocular. *Logos: Revista de Lingüística, Filosofía y Literatura, 31*(1), 202–217.

El-Fattah, A. (2021). *You Have Not Yet Been Defeated: Selected Works 2011–2021.* Fitzcarraldo Editions.

Fernback, J. (2013). Sousveillance: Communities of Resistance to the Surveillance Environment. *Telematics and Informatics, 30*(1), 11–21.

Gordon-Zolov, T., & Zolov, E. (2022). *The Walls of Santiago: Social Revolution and Political Aesthetics in Contemporary Chile.* Berghahn Books.

Herrera, L. (2014). *Revolution in the Age of Social Media: The Egyptian Insurrection and the Internet*. Verso.

INDH. (2019). *Informe Anual: Situación de los Derechos Humanos en Chile 2019, 17 de Octubre - 30 de Noviembre 2019.* INDH.

Inter-American Commission on Human Rights. (2022). *Situación de Derechos Humanos en Chile.* IACHR.

Kornbluh, A. (2024). *Immediacy, or The Style of Too Late Capitalism.* Verso.

Kozman, C. (2023). Alternative Media and Digital Platforms: Empowerment Tools for Civic Engagement. In J. Karam & R. Majed (Eds.), *The Lebanon Uprising of 2019: Voices from the Revolution.* I.B. Tauris.

Lacan, J. (1998). *The Seminar of Jacques Lacan, Book XI: The Four Fundamental Concepts of Psychoanalysis.* W. W. Norton & Company.

Landaeta, L., & Herrero, V. (2021). *La Revuelta. Las Semanas de Octubre que Estremecieron Chile*. Editorial Planeta.

Meruane, L. (2021). *Zona Ciega*. Random House.

Mortensen, M., Neumayer, C., & Poell, T. (Eds.). (2019). *Social Media Materialities and Protest: Critical Reflections*. Routledge.

5

The Fantasy of Impotence

In her study of the emotional experience of embracing social change, Hannah Proctor (2024) shows how this process is almost endemically accompanied by contradictory dynamics. She puts forward the notion of 'asynchronicity' to capture the fact that social and psychic transformation rarely move at the same pace. For her, the history of left-wing political defeats over the past centuries demonstrates that when social change is underway, we cannot help but to feel out of sync—as if we, individually, lag behind transformation. The psychic toll of fighting for social change is therefore not solely ascribed to the oppressive systems that are being challenged, but also to the tempo of transformation itself. Our position within progressive and radical movements, socialist experiments, and contemporary revolts has historically proven difficult to sustain, in large part because change gives rise to opposing logics, mutually incompatible orientations, and seemingly ambivalent forces that cannot be fully reconciled. One thing is to be sure that ours is the time for change; it is quite another to be sure that we are keeping time with change.

The *estallido* was no exception. Disorientation is arguably the most apt term to describe how Chileans felt in the wake of the popular uprising.

G. Sánchez, *A Rebel Unconscious*, Studies in the Psychosocial, https://doi.org/10.1007/978-3-032-12275-9_5

As a journalist put it in his chronicle: 'Over these four months, the *estallido* has been festivity, communion, reflection, barbarism, delinquency, and war' (Fernández, 2020, p. 13). A single day could be painted with all these hues. As a result, a crucial aspect of experiencing the end of neoliberalism was the abrupt introduction of significant degrees of uncertainty into dimensions of quotidian life that had previously been taken for granted. Some of the people I interviewed told me that something as mundane as leaving their homes had become a predicament, as they lived in areas cordoned off by the police. Others did not know whether they would be able to visit family in another city, given that some motorways were completely closed. And even more dramatically, some parents feared not being able to get their children's prescriptions, since nearly all businesses in the city centres were closed, looted, or destroyed. The revolt allowed us to live neoliberalism according to the logic of post-neoliberalism, and that implied infusing bewilderment into everyday life.

The discussion below focuses on a particular way in which the experience of everyday life during the revolt came to harbour opposing dynamics at once. In addition to examining the unconscious dimensions of identifying with social change, the previous chapters have helped to contextualise something rather obvious: the *estallido* compelled people to act continuously. They were engaged in multiple activities at once, from taking part in demonstrations and organising forums, to developing new forms of solidarity among neighbours and providing medical and legal aid to protesters. It is fair to say that terms such as 'inactive' or 'passive' could not be readily applied to most people during the revolt. Yet, as Henri Lefebvre (2014, p. 43) noted, everyday life is defined by contradiction and ambiguity; the most trivial things are often the strangest, as they weave together 'illusion and truth, power and helplessness, the intersection of the sector man controls and the sector he does not control'. In a curious turn, and against the backdrop of this unceasing activity, many of the people I interviewed described themselves as inactive during the *estallido*—what was happening was so overwhelming that they remained immobile. The key point is that they depicted themselves as passive or incapable of acting while simultaneously offering substantial evidence of how effectively they had in fact managed to act. How should we approach this contradiction?

The activity they discursively withdrew from matters here. These were scholars who claimed that, during the uprising, they could not write. While this retreat is justified in intricate and singular ways, it is important to situate both this activity and its absence within a broader cultural context. Researchers have characterised neoliberalism as a regime that distributes the capacity to be capable, so to speak. While the figure of the entrepreneurial subject—who aspires to improve every aspect of their life in order to maximise returns, since they are their own company—is predicated on the ideal of high performance (Bröckling, 2015; Dardot & Laval, 2017), it has also been noted that neoliberalism also directly produces incapable bodies. For Jasbir Puar (2017), neoliberalism increases the demand for bodily capacity but, at the same time, renders such a goal unattainable. This creates a political economy where 'all bodies are being evaluated in relation to their success or failure in terms of health, wealth, progressive productivity, upward mobility, enhanced capacity' (p. 15). In a culture of performance and capable bodies, succumbing to inactivity and passivity amounts to a failed subject.

The experiences I centre on come from individuals who work at the university, an environment that has been extensively portrayed as fomenting this performance culture (Ball, 2003; Leyton & Sánchez, 2024; Morrissey, 2015). In the midst of the neoliberal passion for excellence, permanent improvement, and capable bodies, not writing could be seen as a way of ignoring the injunction to perform—that is, as an act of resistance by embracing the experience of the end of neoliberalism. And yet, they did write. When narrating their experiences, their activity was made admissible only through a substitute, which is precisely the definition of the symptom in psychoanalysis. The symptom is a surrogate formation that implies a certain non-knowledge on the part of the subject (Žižek, 2008). Unbearable situations can become psychically manageable insofar as something else stands in, allowing for a roundabout access to them without the subject consciously knowing it. From this angle, the contradiction of proclaiming an inability to write during the revolt while nevertheless exerting this capacity becomes the site of unconscious investments—investments that can offer further insight into the desire for social change.

As my interpretation will demonstrate, the capacity/debility divide at the core of the political economy of our control societies (Puar, 2017) has its own libidinal economy. The *estallido* conspicuously illustrates this. While it is undeniable that neoliberalism has evolved into a biopolitical regime that unequally distributes capacity and debility across populations, this alone tells us little about how we come to be recognised as capable or debilitated subjects—or why, during the revolt, capacity at times had to be camouflaged as its opposite. Perhaps we should take this as an index of our irreducibility to historically determined subject positions and, crucially, of the symbolic mediation of our desire. By accepting that the priority in our desire is not its object but the obstacle, the overlap between activity and passivity during the uprising challenges the capacity/debility dyad and the analytic primacy attributed to bodily matter. Since humans have a conflicted relationship with their own desires, 'an unconscious part of them is prepared to ignore reality, deny logic and expect satisfaction against all odds and at all costs' (Bailly, 2023, p. 855). From this perspective, we make room for an interpretation of the counterintuitive idea that we might desire impotence.

Can We Do Nothing?

The disorientation generated by the *estallido* can be perceived in the recurring claim among interviewees that they suddenly 'did not know' things—basic things, taken-for-granted aspects of everyday life. It is as though the readability of their world had abruptly collapsed. Many interviews ooze a sense of existential or vital perplexity stemming from the sudden disruption of routine life; people no longer knew how to carry on with their most prosaic pursuits. The revolt interrupted the continuity of ordinary tasks—cooking, commuting, taking children to school—which became overlaid with uncertainty and unpredictability. The street, usually a traversable and intelligible space, was now described as a site of contingency and danger, a space where you 'didn't know what you would find'. This is what Manuel Canales (2022) refers to as the break in the neoliberal normalcy of Chileans' everyday life. Or, as the philosopher Aïcha Messina (2020, p. 9) laconically put it in the preface of her book—whose launch was delayed by the revolt: 'What has happened since 18 October is that the city is suspended'. The ambiguity of this term is, in fact, appropriate: it conveys both a temporary halt to activity and the sense that things were almost hanging in the air.

This sense of suspension can be felt in most publications on the revolt. While the anti-neoliberal character of the uprising is never questioned—not even in the most phlegmatic analyses (e.g., Peña & Silva, 2022)—there is also a recurring acknowledgement of the difficulties involved in writing about it. The feminist philosopher Alejandra Castillo (2019, p. 64) described this as follows: 'It is because of this acceleration and incompleteness that any analysis of the revolt can only take the form of a chronicle (a testimony, an opinion or reaction) whose narrative unfolds more in the day-to-day than in theoretical pretensions'. The nature of the uprising destabilises the very possibility of its analysis; translating the events into words inevitably felt like a formidable task. Similarly, in his book on the *estallido*, the philosopher Rodrigo Karmy (2019, p. 15) defined his writing as 'sketches'; provisional, exploratory, and insufficient materials that attempt to convey a force that they cannot properly contain. 'Their conditions of production', Karmy continues, 'were bound to the various moments of the Chilean revolt, which cut through the writing as if a storm had swept over thought'. Since the *estallido* cut through the writing, it is no surprise that most publications present themselves as 'notes' or 'fragments'—pieces that do not complete a puzzle.

The revolt posed a quandary for critical scholars, one that was particularly acute during the first months of its unfolding. If we lend credence to the idea that 'to critique is to wish for and work toward change', as Kristin Ross (2023, p. 101) maintains, the principal channel for this has traditionally been academic writing—or writing performed by academics, which is not necessarily the same. The *estallido*, one of the most profound experiences of social change ever to occur in the country, nevertheless, turned writing into a daunting task. The case of Cristina, a social sciences scholar, vividly captures these difficulties. The following is an excerpt from when she began to describe her everyday life during October and November 2019:

> I didn't do anything; I didn't do anything because I considered that nothing was worthwhile. I mean, one couldn't pretend that nothing was happening, so I did nothing. I devoted myself to painting a wall in my house, which was the only thing I could do. It was unbearable, the anxiety was really unbearable, it was unbearable [...]. I remember perfectly – I could even send you some pictures of the wall if you want. They were some little drawings; I used an insole for that, and I painted them with a brush – with a tiny brush! I waited for it to dry a little to take the insole out so that it wouldn't get stained. I dried it with the hairdryer and put it back on. So, it took me, I don't know, man, like five days [to complete it]. So, yeah, I did very little – I did very, very little. Now, all in all, I don't know how, I don't know how I've got like five things [academic articles]. Every year I get like five or eight publications, and I'm like, "where from?" I don't know where they came from, but even at that moment when I did nothing, something happened.

Many aspects of this fragment are worth underscoring. Cristina's interviews were among the most challenging, as the *estallido* left an indelible mark on her—a mark shaped by helplessness. On several occasions, especially when her speech drew near to sorrowful memories, she remarked that she did not remember things very well. Her account constantly oscillated between not recalling certain events and not wanting to recall them. Interestingly, however, painting a wall in her house is something she remembers 'perfectly'. Numerous factors could be at play in interpreting the appeal of this recollection, but one could argue that it has something to do with counterposing the activeness of painting against what she experienced as the inactiveness of the revolt. According to her, the situation was unbearable as all she could do was wait; activity was only possible for those on the barricades or in political negotiations, and she took part in neither—although she was present on the streets, she steered clear of combative action. Consequently, Cristina found herself in a situation she could not inhabit, an impossibility. Yet instead of going out, where activity lay for her, she remained indoors.

At first glance, her narration could be placed alongside many other examples of uncertainty during the revolt. Just as others did not know how to move across the city, what to expect on the streets, or when public transport would be operative again, Cristina did not know how she had managed to write academic articles in the wake of the uprising. The way in which activity and passivity meet in her speech, however, offers us an important interpretive clue. Cristina's account of her everyday life during the revolt is consonant with the logic of symbolic satisfaction, exemplified by Lacan through the anorexic experience. Lacan proposed that when the satisfaction of a need is replaced by a symbolic type of satisfaction, it is not enough to say that the real, concrete object has been conferred the status of a symbol. What truly matters, he insists, is that both the symbolic value and accent lie in the field of activity, since it is the 'mode of apprehension'—and not the object itself—that is granted a symbolic character. Such a character is the result of the eroticisation of an activity: the libidinal wrapping of something that, through its recursiveness, provides a satisfaction that is not imprinted in the activity itself. Lacan's point is that, when it comes to object relations, objects are important yet not crucial—what is crucial is what we do with them.

In order to demonstrate this point, Lacan goes as far as to suggest that symbolic satisfaction can be obtained even when no real object is at stake. For him, only this can explain a symptom like anorexia. To place emphasis on the object itself would obscure what is psychically at issue: it is not simply that the anorexic subject does not eat anything, but rather that the subject actively eats 'nothing'. And that is possible because 'nothing' exists within the symbolic register so it can, in effect, be eaten. Eating nothing is not the same as the negation of eating; it is a symbolic activity in its own right. Symbolic satisfaction can thus be derived from the act: 'From this savoured absence as such, he [the anorexic] makes use of what he has in front of him, namely the mother on whom he depends. In virtue of this nothing, he makes her dependent on him' (Lacan, 2020, p. 177).

With the above as background, let me now go over Cristina's sequential claims at the beginning of the quotation: (a) I didn't do anything, (b) I considered that nothing was worthwhile, (c) one couldn't pretend that nothing was happening, (d) I did nothing. It is hard to find a more resolute way of expressing her conscious relinquishment of activity. Nevertheless, when read from a strictly symbolic perspective—where 'nothing' actually exists as a thing—the progression of her speech hints at a content beyond her intended meaning.

> Moment 1: The emphasis is on the negation of an activity, namely, the fact that she did not do anything. Consciously, no object was part of her pursuits. However, the way in which this is phrased admits another association. 'I didn't do anything' can also suggest that she did not simply engage in just anything or whatever, but rather that she partook in something more specific, albeit still undetermined.
> Moment 2: Cristina shifts from 'anything' to 'nothing' in order to substantiate her conscious attempt to cease being active. Given the context, 'nothing was worthwhile' appears as an admission of the futility of engaging in activities that once felt meaningful – on reflection, every endeavour seemed pointless. From a different angle, this can also be read as a realisation: 'nothing', this symbolic piece, became 'worthwhile' – that is, a valued element in Cristina's symbolic world.
> Moment 3: Cristina seems to further stress the futility of action by claiming it was impossible to turn a blind eye to the situation on the street. The magnitude of the events was so immense that they could no longer be ignored, so 'one couldn't pretend that nothing was happening'. Looking outside was enough to realise that nothing was all you could do. Once again, an alternative reading of her speech emerges: 'nothing' not only became a valuable symbolic element, but now 'nothing' was literally taking place in front of her eyes – to the extent that it became impossible for her to pretend otherwise. In the wake of the uprising, something she deemed worthwhile was now happening, and she could not disguise her interest.
> Moment 4: Finally, in a context in which 'nothing' holds a precious symbolic status and demands attention, she decided to actively partake in it; she started to *do nothing*.

From a literal reading of Cristina's speech—intended to show me that she refrained from activity—it becomes clear that things were very different at the unconscious level. The fragment I interpreted reveals how closely intertwined activity and passivity were during the revolt: unconscious activity was registered under the guise of conscious passivity. She wrote several articles, but this came out as a surprise, given that all she consciously acknowledged was a withdrawal from activity. It can be said that Cristina invested herself in an unconscious nothing-as-activity in order to overcome the conscious nothing-as-passivity that the *estallido* brought for her. When seen through the logic of symbolic satisfaction, she unconsciously eroticised 'nothing' to regain a sense of control over the situation: *nothing was happening*, an event beyond her volitional, conscious mastery, so she unconsciously decided to cease being passive by *doing nothing*. The libidinisation of 'nothing' allowed her to engineer an unconscious mode of being in a context where many simply could not consciously afford to be. Her case shows us that, at least psychically, it is rather difficult to do nothing.

Accepting that symbolic satisfaction derives primarily from the subject's activity should not, however, lead us to think that the singularity of the objects involved in this dynamic is wholly unimportant. Of all things, Cristina chose to placate the anxiety induced by what was happening by painting a wall in her house. She insinuates that this was a rather meaningless thing to do—and this is precisely why it can be portrayed as doing nothing, as something that *does not count* as being active in the context of the revolt. Therefore, painting is a consciously insignificant activity that is in solidarity with her unconscious 'doing nothing'. Among the aspects that come to the fore in her description is the painstaking nature of the activity she chose to undertake. It was not simply a matter of changing the colour of a wall or renovating a washed-out surface. Cristina engaged in a meticulous, cumbersome task: she painted 'small patterns' that required 'tiny brushes', and in order to proceed, she had to wait 'a little bit' to move the insole. Everything appeared to be on a miniature scale and highly time-consuming because, as she declares, she wanted to kill as much time as possible.

When we put her activity-that-is-not-activity in context, was she not replicating indoors what was happening outdoors? As I showed in the previous chapters, the walls on the street were a privileged vehicle for the interpellation of the Other of the *estallido*. Cristina felt that all she could do was reproduce on her walls what the demonstrators were doing on the streets. 'Chile woke up', 'neoliberalism was born and will die in Chile', and 'until dignity becomes habit' are some of the mottoes that were scrawled across the public space. Cristina, for whom action was beyond her reach, revamped her walls with little drawings painted with tiny brushes. We can see how the parallel with the anorexic experience is particularly fortunate. For Lacan, the anorexic turns the tables on her symbolic dependency: by attaining unconscious satisfaction from a 'savoured absence', the subject attempts to exert control over the Other in order to manage her dependence on it. Similarly, Cristina found unconscious satisfaction in her 'passive activity', as this allowed her to regain mastery over the events—by perceiving herself as completely at the mercy of the Other, she succeeded in making everything depend on her (in)activity. Her painting was dainty, punctilious, and dilatory simply because she was in charge.

'Even at that moment when I did nothing, something happened' is how the vignette concludes. She acknowledged that the *estallido* was calling Chileans—that is why she could not pretend that nothing was happening—and her response was to let it ring, as it were. Her passivity in the face of the interpellation of the Other was an unconscious way of having the upper hand, allowing her to carry on business as usual in other areas of her life. Her sense of awe when accounting for the seemingly inexplicable fact that she maintained an impressive publishing track while deserting from activity is genuine, since her activity was not consciously registered—or, to be precise, because she was unconsciously active. This becomes less of a mystery when we approach her speech from the perspective of symbolic satisfaction. Just as 'seeing everything' opened up the libidinal economy of the fantasy of immediacy, here 'doing nothing' proves, at times, to be the best way to achieve what we want.

Doing What You Can't

This atypical situation, in which capacity is somehow made to coalesce with its opposite, is expressed again in the case of Carlos, an interdisciplinary scholar. His speech epitomises the strange amalgamation of activity and passivity also discernible in Cristina's. Unlike most interviews, his narration was organised from the outset around academic labour. Furthermore, much of the conversation was guided by the weight he gives to the idea that 'the revolt meant that a large part of the academic world had to recognise and confront its own impotence'. Obliquely insinuated by Cristina, now the signifier 'impotence' openly orients Carlos' speech.

> What happened was that [the revolt] revealed that, from within academia, not much can be said or done about the situation, because we were completely overwhelmed by it, right? We were completely overwhelmed by something that we already knew could, sooner or later, extend into a future entirely removed from our experience – that is, looking far ahead, it was going to happen sooner or later, you know? Sooner or later, sooner or later.

The term he deploys in Spanish, '*desbordado*', has a similar semantic depth to 'overwhelmed' in English. Both imply, simultaneously, an external overflowing that produces a sense of defeat, and the state in which someone is seized by a sudden, strong emotion. 'Overwhelmed' was a term many interviewees drew on during my fieldwork, often with deep despondency. This is another example of the disorientation produced by the rupture in the flow of everyday life. If we take the quotidian to be 'what happens when nothing happens' (Giannini, 1987, p. 21), we can see that the revolt made something happen which, regardless of its desirability, was not easily endured. Interestingly, this very term has been used to describe the *estallido*. According to Nelly Richard (2021, p. 57), the revolt was 'a utopian overflow [*desborde*] expressing the desire to change everything'. Carlos was inhabiting this utopian overflow, this desire to change everything, with a sharp sense of impotence.

Let us return to his description of the events. What exactly is that 'something' bound to happen, which was responsible for the overwhelming tenor of the situation? An initial reading suggests that the sentence refers to the *estallido* itself; the revolt was destined to happen sooner or later. Following the onset of the uprising, much of the local academic debate quickly came to centre on a peculiar divide: those who purportedly saw the revolt coming, and those who did not.[1] In simple terms, one could only be either on the side of enlightenment or on the side of ignorance. Carlos appears to be alluding to this debate. The sentence is, however, just imprecise enough to permit a slightly alternative reading: what if that 'something' was the acknowledgement of academia's impotence? This offers a possible way of interpreting the otherwise puzzling line about how this 'something' might be extended 'into a future entirely removed from our experience'. The idea that the *estallido* could be something removed from our Chilean experience seems difficult to endorse—the revolt, if anything, is precisely one of those events from which subjects cannot subtract themselves. An impotent academic activity, conversely, is something that can indeed be extended indefinitely.

Impotence is an intriguing thing though. Carlos' realisation came after the publication of an essay he had contributed to a collective book on the *estallido*. The book was launched in early March 2020, almost five months after the revolt began. Afterwards, he briefly entertained the idea of expanding the arguments presented in that piece into a full-length book of his own, although he told me that this idea withered away quickly. For him, it was simply not possible. 'This impossibility', Carlos points out, 'was precisely the effect of what was happening; it wasn't the time to start writing'. This perception is accompanied by an important addition: the others who wrote nonetheless.

> And, well, there were people in "academia" who, of course, jumped the gun […], they all had two books immediately written at the time, which gave a very strange image – also a very grotesque one, as it reinforced that idea of intellectual writing coming from an ivory tower. Although that wasn't necessarily the case, it created that impression, and one would say: "Well, what would someone completely outside of this see?" […] That's what it came to mean for me over time, and that's why I couldn't write in the end; it wasn't even a decision but something that simply happened that way, as though I was paralysed – there was a kind of paralysis, yeah.

[1] Hence, Danilo Martuccelli's (2019, p. 371) caveat that any analysis of the *estallido* must first 'set aside both the sincere naïveté of those who admit they did not see this coming, and the dubious apocalyptic certainties of those who always knew it would'.

> And what happened, I think, was precisely the revelation, over time, quite immediately, of a kind of impotence.

There are multiple aspects I would like to highlight from this vignette. Firstly, a sort of paralysis is once again attributed to the *estallido*, just as in Cristina's case. And once again, this reference is pervaded by tensions. The discursive collusion between movement and inactivity emerges in Carlos' speech in a rather blatant way. He conveyed to me a strong sense of satisfaction with the piece he wrote for the collective book yet, in the same breath he claimed, decisively, that 'it wasn't the time to start writing'. The irony of all this is that he reached the conclusion that writing in the midst of the *estallido* was impossible by writing an article on the *estallido* while it was happening. In other words, Carlos realised that he could not do something because he had, in fact, already done it.

The unfolding of Carlos' speech goes even further. As noted above, he constructs a transgressive other. In a first movement, he distances himself from certain academics who do not properly belong—or should not belong—to the academic realm. He accomplishes this manoeuvre by using quotation marks during our interview when referring to those people in 'academia'. In a second movement, the same people are singled out as part of a group of scholars who acted prematurely, all too hastily when it came to saying something about the *estallido*. Although he asserts that the problem lies in how much these interventions helped to reinforce the familiar perception that academics are normally detached from pedestrian events—since they write from the top of their ivory towers—there are other, more subtle elements at play. The notions of 'decision' and 'immediacy' seem to be pointing to something significant—something Carlos is not saying directly about his own attachment to academic writing.

Let me momentarily put a pin in the fact that Carlos did write about the *estallido* during the *estallido*. Taken literally, his denunciation of what the others did echoes the Wittgensteinian adage: 'Whereof one cannot speak, thereof one must be silent'.[2] The same strange prohibition of an

[2] In the Routledge edition of the *Tractatus*, it reads: 'The whole sense of the book might be summed up in the following words: what can be said at all can be said clearly, and what we cannot talk about we must pass over in silence' (Wittgenstein, 2002, p. 3).

impossible task seems to be at stake in Carlos' speech. Writing about the *estallido* while it was unfolding was an activity that, on the one hand, could not be carried out and, on the other, had to be ruled out since people could nonetheless jump the gun. This prohibition seems to be breached by the instantaneous exercise of willpower on the part of the others. These others 'had two books *immediately* written at the time', while for him, the impossibility of writing 'wasn't even a decision but something that simply happened that way'. And for Carlos, all this manifested as 'the revelation, over time, quite *immediately*, of a kind of impotence'. Two interesting additions emerge here. First, while making comparisons with the others, Carlos felt the need to emphasise that, for him, it wasn't *even* a decision; it did not actually reach that threshold—whereas for the others, it seems legitimate to infer, it was entirely volitional from the outset. Second, he corrects himself in the very last line by affirming that the revelation of the impotence did not happen over time but rather 'quite immediately'. My suggestion is that these are important features to understand Carlos' fantasmatic scaffolding here.

To be sure, I am not trying to determine here whether writing during the revolt was right or wrong. What I am trying to do is make sense of the following sequence: Carlos wrote a piece, only to retroactively realise that writing was no longer possible, he subsequently condemned those who immediately decided to do what was not possible, and finally he reached the conclusion that there was a sense of impotence within academia. Once we remove the pin from the fact that Carlos did write an article—much like the others did—the following question demands an answer: what differentiates these two kinds of writing? My suggestion is that what makes the whole libidinal difference for him is his awareness of the impotence of academia. True, Carlos did exactly what he criticises the others for, yet he places himself in a different position. The others had books fully written *immediately*, whereas he could not even make the decision to write, because the revelation of academia's impotence came to him *immediately*. His knowledge is the reason why his own text is not registered in his speech as a breach of the rule—as he stated in the previous quote, he was overwhelmed by something he 'already knew'. If the *estallido* revealed the impotence of academia, as he claims it did, then

Carlos' knowledge distanced him from (the enjoyment of) such impotence. He seems to rely on a fantasy in which a supposed other enjoys improperly—in a way he would not allow himself to—so his writing is not part of the same libidinal economy.

The interpretation I offer is less far-fetched than it may initially appear. Certainly, impotence does not present itself as an appealing condition to be consciously subjected to. The point is that we are not dealing here, primarily, with impotence as a kind of practical unfitness or incapacity, but rather with impotence as a libidinally charged scenario. As Žižek (2008) maintains, the Other is not simply the network of rules and presuppositions upon which our speech activity is grounded; it also entails a series of permitted transgressions against these rules and presuppositions. The Other has a more or less clandestine face, an obscene support that, far from undermining its alleged solidity, grants the possibility for group cohesion. 'Impotence', I propose, is the signifier that allows Carlos to stage a complex fantasmatic scenario of transgressions: both those performed by the others and his own. The others, these quote-unquote academics, congregate around a corrupt enjoyment insofar as they *ought to know* that 'from within academia not much can be said or done about the situation', yet they ignore this, and that is why they wrote. They 'choose' to write because they remain oblivious to their impotence and, for Carlos, that grants them access to a satisfaction inaccessible to him. He knows better than those 'academics'—impotence is no surprise to him—and this gives his article a different imaginary status: it is not a testament to his impotence but evidence that his knowledge holds impotence in place.

Carlos' fantasy follows the logic of fetishism. Freud (2001) claims that the fetish is designed to preserve something from extinction. For him, the primary function of the fetish is to serve as a substitute for a belief: the mother's penis that the little boy used to believe in but does not want to relinquish despite the evidence. The reason is that, if the mother does not have a penis, the little boy assumes that his own is in danger. A substitute is thus needed to prevent castration henceforth. The singularity of the logic of the fetish—the disavowal—is that what is refuted is simultaneously acknowledged: 'In the conflict between the weight of the unwelcome perception and the force of his counter-wish, a compromise has been reached, as is only possible under the dominance of the unconscious laws of thought' (Freud, 2001, p. 154). Following this logic, the fantasy of impotence allows Carlos to retain the belief that he is not part of the academia that writes about the revolt *because he knows better than the others*. As his experience shows, sustaining these mutually incompatible assertions requires strong libidinal investments.

What the experiences of Cristina and Carlos clearly show is how academic writing lost its taken-for-grantedness during the revolt. This might explain the imaginary lengths they need to go to in order to safeguard their attachments to this activity and so regain subjective consistency. Their speeches are beset with tensions, breaches, contradictions, and exceptions that speak volumes about the unconscious impact of the call of the *estallido*. This is particularly evident in the case of Carlos. He and his colleagues did the exact same thing—they wrote about the revolt while it was still happening—and yet he feels the pressure to detach himself from this activity by creating a convoluted fantasmatic scenario of passivity. Given that all of them proved equally capable of producing texts, it is hard to say that they were factually impotent. None of this, however, prevents impotence from playing a fantasmatic role. Ultimately, it all boils down to what the participants know: Carlos knows academics are impotent, that they cannot write; he and the other academics wrote nonetheless, yet his awareness of impotence separates his writing from theirs. The others might not even suspect they are impotent, but he knows. Carlos appears to be very aware that what is impossible should be forbidden, since its transgression is highly enjoyable.

Sacrificing Knowledge

By the end of the decade of mass protests, the Italian philosopher Franco Berardi (2019) published *Futurability*, a book with the disquieting subtitle *The Age of Impotence and the Horizon of Possibility*. The age of impotence described by Berardi is the outcome of decades of neoliberalism's privatisation of what he calls the general intellect. In his view, social knowledge is the source of workers' autonomy, but this emancipatory potential has been captured by the neoliberal counter-revolution and redirected towards the service of economic accumulation. The general intellect possesses the potency—understood as a form of subjective energy—to actualise the possibilities inscribed in the current composition of the world and, in doing so, transform it in an emancipatory direction. Yet the cognitive automation and endless connectivity upon which the global economy relies have resulted in 'the impotence of subjectivity' (p. 21). For Berardi, this impotence is a symptom of disproportion: the fact that reason can no longer govern the hyper-connectivity in which we live. Amid the inertia of possibilities induced by neoliberalism, there remains a capacity to unlock new horizons: 'Beyond impotence and power [...], knowledge is the social dimension where the bad dream of capitalism can be dispelled at last: not simply reversed, I mean wholly abandoned as an empty space, forgotten as a nightmare' (p. 197).

Through knowledge, we will regain our collective potency. This, in turn, will allow us to leave behind our impotent subjectivity and awaken from the bad dream of capitalism. Although I would very much like to believe that, at least part of the experience of the *estallido* does not conform to this description. Berardi's approach to knowledge is embedded in an immanent theory of possibilities that must, however, exclude one possibility: negativity. Non-coincidence, lack of self-identity, structural alienation—in a word, the unconscious—has no role to play in the configuration of the impotent subjectivity he attributes to neoliberalism. This necessary omission helps explain why, for Berardi, impotence is invariably something undesirable; impotent is something we must certainly do not want to be.[3] In his view, the potency of the general

[3] Berardi's book on the unconscious only confirms this. Drawing on Deleuze and Guattari, he treats the unconscious as a 'creative potency' rather than as the product of our symbolic dependency. This aligns his approach more closely with a kind of aesthetic unconscious: 'a laboratory of cutting and pasting, a laboratory of dance, of syntonization with the rhythm of chaos' (Berardi, 2021, p. 65). Since structural alienation and enjoyment have no place in his conception of the unconscious, Berardi can close his book wholeheartedly perplexed by the 'incomprehensible' stubbornness of humans who engage in actions long proven to be failures. One is left wishing that someone had conceptualised a way of gaining satisfaction beyond the bounds of pleasure.

intellect was impounded by an external force, but this only reinforces the positive status of knowledge—knowledge and the general intellect coincide, unless something obstructs their union. Were we to adopt Berardi's perspective, the experiences of Cristina and Carlos would remain unintelligible, as not rebelling against impotence during the revolt would be inconceivable. However, once we factor in the rebelliousness of the unconscious, impotence is not necessarily a curtailment of our potency.

The logic of fetishism gives us an answer. As mentioned, for Freud the fetish functions as a peculiar defensive mechanism: in order to retain a belief without which we would fall apart, the fetish enables us to preserve the effect of that belief even while acknowledging its failure. So, it is not that the little boy represses the disturbing memory of seeing nothing where he expected something, but rather that he acknowledges his mother does not have a penis and *this very acknowledgement* allows him to carry on believing that she does. Through Lacan's conceptualisation of castration as a symbolic experience, the logic of fetish can be understood as an unconscious mechanism for dealing with the lack of the Other—that is, the fact that I cannot attain self-recognition because the entity that should secure this process is itself incomplete. Therefore, the logic of the fetish operates differently from the 'I do not want to know anything about X' of repression. Disavowal is the process of the fetishist. Alenka Zupančič (2024) has offered a topological description of this. Repression requires two levels: our reality and another dimension to which the repressed memory is consigned so that it cannot disrupt that reality. Disavowal, by contrast, is one-dimensional—the disruptive element remains entirely within our reality. Nothing is made to disappear; rather, what disturbs us has changed its disturbing character through the fetish.

'I know very well, but nonetheless...' is the formula of disavowal (see Mannoni, 2003). I know very well that my mum does not have a penis, but nonetheless I conduct my life as if she does. The fantasy of impotence I reconstructed in this chapter follows the same logic: I know very well that I wrote articles like everyone else, but nonetheless I will pretend that I did not. Neither Cristina nor Carlos attempted to repress the existence of their writings; quite the opposite, they acknowledged and openly spoke about their articles. These texts are entirely part of their reality, but they were imaginarily transformed. Their capacity was turned into incapacity through a laborious unconscious operation. My point is that it would be an interpretive mistake to dismiss this as a nonsensical move. Why go to the trouble of disavowing their acts instead of simply accepting what their own speech already acknowledges? Because this manoeuvre affords them the imaginary ability to preserve the integrity of the Other of the *estallido*. Through their disavowals, the ambiguity of the Other's call ceases to be a source of anxiety. Why? Because, by virtue of their knowing, they were now the ones calling the shots.[4]

Jack Black (2025) suggests that cynical disavowal is the unconscious mechanism in which what is strictly disavowed is knowledge. The cynical position rests on a self-perceived enlightenment: cynics not only know, but they know better than everyone else. This stance enables cynics to distance themselves from their own knowledge, to disavow it. Crucially, they transgress the rule *only to uphold the authority of the Other*. They recognise that the Other is lacking, that recognition cannot be attained through its call, so they adopt a posture of nonconformity in order to reinforce the Law. Carlos' experience clearly follows this logic. He does not stop at the acknowledgement of impotence; he goes further by discursively reprimanding the '(bad) academics' for breaking the rules by writing. His own texts lie outside this sphere of misdemeanour because he 'immediately' knew such an act was not permissible, so he effectively *sacrificed his better knowledge* for the sake of preserving the enjoyment of the Other. He did write, claimed that this was not possible, and displayed evidence of his writing because this is how he unconsciously negotiated the lack in the Other of the *estallido*. His transgression made him an instrument in the service of the Law of the Other, but also rendered the Other dependent on his superior knowledge.

[4] This unconscious dimension is entirely overlooked in approaches to disavowal that treat it merely as a particular speech act. Grace Paterson (2023), for example, takes disavowal as a way for a speaker to distance themselves from past speech acts without implying a full retraction. It is, for her, a mode of language use with distinct characteristics. She acknowledges that it is possible to wholly deny agency over an action, but these are 'instances of extreme impairment and loss of control, such as sleepwalking and psychosis' (p. 339). Such individuals are, in her view, 'genuinely alienated' from the action; however, she regards these as rare and exceptional cases. What is not admissible here is the unconscious use of disavowal precisely as a mechanism to manage an encounter with alienation.

At the end of the day, disavowal requires a tremendous amount of psychic movement for one to remain in the same place. It functions as an unconscious mechanism to avoid an encounter with the transformative dimension of knowledge. As Black puts it, the cynic establishes a manipulative distance from its own knowledge to continue desiring. In this sense, we can openly admit that the *estallido* transformed everything—that it made us impotent—yet knowledge provides the means to remain intact by sacrificing that very knowledge. Within the fantasy of impotence, one can simultaneously accept the radical transformation brought about by the revolt and remain unfazed by the events. We can now perceive the gulf separating this unconscious use of knowledge to sustain impotence from Berardi's affirmation that knowledge serves as a cure for impotent subjectivity. In Carlos' account, there are no external machinations or power structures seeking to limit our potency; the revolt itself rendered us impotent. And yet, when confronted with the emancipatory call of the Other of the *estallido*, Carlos turned his knowledge into a fetish—thereby conceding the transformative potential of the revolt, while carrying on desiring as usual. Far from Berardi's overly optimistic view, the fantasy of impotence shows that we are willing to sacrifice knowledge for unconscious satisfaction.

We have arrived at another way of unconsciously responding to the call of the *estallido*. As with the fantasy of sleeplessness, in the fantasy of impotence the subject is confronted with the impossibility of responding to this call. In this case, however, there is no direct identification with the Other, but rather a kind of tug of war between the subject and the Other. The subject does not repress castration—on the contrary, it is fully aware of it—but throws this knowledge into the Other's kiln to keep it burning. As Carlos' experience demonstrates so pristinely, what he wants is to see the Other remain operative. His transgression serves a way of verifying the Other's existence, to put it to work. The crucial point is that *he makes it work*, so castration becomes now co-dependence. A similar dynamic is at play in Cristina's case. She made everything conditional on her passivity—she 'did nothing' by placidly engaging in a meticulous activity unconsciously designed to keep the Other alert. What these responses reveal is an inability to tolerate even a slight dent in their modes of enjoyment. Everything can be transformed so long as I can continue to extract unconscious satisfaction from my activity in the way I always have.

My interpretation corroborates something that psychoanalysis has long maintained: far from being what informs our will to act—whether in a retrograde or an emancipatory direction—knowledge can serve as the medium through which things appear to be moving, even as we continue with business as usual. As the fantasy of impotence demonstrates, disavowal is an unconscious mechanism whose psychic appeal lies in the incorporation of defiance into the very structure of fantasising. I know how things are—I know *very well* that social change is underway—and yet I am willing to sacrifice this precious knowledge for the sake of my unconscious satisfaction. 'The sacrifice of one's knowledge through disavowal', McGowan (2022, p. 92) claims, 'increases the libidinal power of the fantasy for the subject'. Disavowal operates in broad daylight, precisely because its aim is to make the Other the subject's hostage. When the Other addresses the subject partially or inconsistently, the subject responds with further sacrifice: unable to tolerate alienation, the subject gives away its knowledge of castration to even out the (in)capacity of the Other.

Trying to be in control of the Other eloquently illustrates that it is much easier to know about change than to allow such knowledge to change us. Through disavowal, we put a great deal of effort into avoiding being struck by this knowledge. Potency, as we can see, is not necessarily what is always at stake. This is precisely what cultural approaches to impotence fail to grasp. In his highly erudite book *Impotence: A Cultural History*, Angus McLaren (2007) convincingly proves that, throughout history, men have spared no effort in their torturous pursuit of restoring their lost potency. Furthermore, this quest has not always carried the same meaning: although inadequacy has historically been perceived as a condition to be corrected, it has not been corrected for the same reasons. The underlying assumption is that male potency can be dulled by different cultural forces, but that every culture strives to sharpen it anew. And how has this been done? Through knowledge. Yet, the experience of the *estallido* presents an alternative picture: without denying the societal pressure to display potency, impotence can be libidinised to the point of becoming extremely potent at a psychic level.

The fantasy of impotence accounts for an imaginary way of appropriating alienation amid the experience of the end of neoliberalism. Alienation is what we invariably received from the Other during the revolt, something Cristina and Carlos were well aware of. The *estallido* brought an experience beyond their control, and their response was not to be transformed by this knowledge but rather to use it to become 'the master of ceremonies of this alienation which, *du coup*, ceases to be operative as alienation' (Zupančič, 2024, p. 77). This fantasmatic framework stages a kind of psychic judo move: the destabilising knowledge coming from the Other is redirected to destabilise the Other in return. The sole problem is that this destabilising knowledge is the emancipatory nucleus of the revolt. Alienation—what made the *estallido* a transformative experience—is turned into an instrument of enjoyment. 'In this precise sense', Zupančič concludes, 'it might be said that castration is used here as a defence against castration' (p. 85). The fantasy of impotence deactivated the transformative knowledge of the revolt by turning it into enjoyment fuel.

References

Bailly, L. (2023). A Lacanian Perspective on Identity. *The International Journal of Psychoanalysis, 104*(5), 855–859.

Ball, S. (2003). The Teacher's Soul and the Terrors of Performativity. *Journal of Education Policy, 18*(2), 215–228.

Berardi, F. (2019). *Futurability*. Verso.

Berardi, F. (2021). *The Third Unconscious*. Verso.

Black, J. (2025). Examining the Mechanism of Disavowal and Its Two Forms: Cynical Disavowal and Fetishistic Disavowal. *Theory & Psychology, 35*(1), 117–135.

Bröckling, U. (2015). *The Entrepreneurial Self: Fabricating a New Type of Subject*. SAGE Publications.

Canales, M. (2022). *La Pregunta de Octubre: Fundación, Apogeo y Crisis del Chile Neoliberal*. LOM Ediciones.

Castillo, A. (2019). *Asamblea de los Cuerpos*. Sangría Editora.
Dardot, P., & Laval, C. (2017). *The New Way of the World: On Neoliberal Society*. Verso.
Fernández, P. (2020). *Sobre la Marcha. Notas Acerca del Estallido Social en Chile*. Debate.
Freud, S. (2001). Fetishism. In *The Standard Edition of the Complete Psychological Works of Sigmund Freud, Vol. XXI (1927–1931)*. Vintage.
Giannini, H. (1987). *La 'Reflexión' Cotidiana*. Editorial Universitaria.
Karmy, R. (2019). *El Porvenir Se Hereda. Fragmentos de un Chile Sublevado*. Sangría Editora.
Lacan, J. (2020). *The Seminar of Jacques Lacan, Book IV: The Object Relation*. Polity.
Lefebvre, H. (2014). *Critique of Everyday Life*. Verso.
Leyton, D., & Sánchez, G. (2024). Beyond (and alongside) Shameful Attachments: The Lived Experience of Critique Within the Entrepreneurial University. *Cultural Studies <=> Critical Methodologies*, *24*(4), 251–262.
Mannoni, O. (2003). 'I Know Well, But All The Same...'. In M. Rothenberg, D. Foster & S. Žižek (Eds.), *Perversion and the Social Relation*. Duke University Press.
Martuccelli, D. (2019). El largo octubre chileno. Bitácora sociológica. In K. Araujo (Ed.), *Hilos Tensados. Para Leer el Octubre Chileno*. Editorial USACH.
McGowan, T. (2022). *The Racist Fantasy: Unconscious Roots of Hatred*. Bloomsbury Academic.
McLaren, A. (2007). *Impotence: A Cultural History*. The University of Chicago Press.
Messina, A. (2020). *Feminismo y Revolución. Crónica de una Inquietud. Santiago 2019, Fragmentos de una Paz Insólita*. Ediciones Metales Pesados.
Morrissey, J. (2015). Regimes of Performance: Practices of the Normalised Self in the Neoliberal University. *British Journal of Sociology of Education, 36* (4), 614–634.
Paterson, G. (2023). On Disavowal. *Topoi: An International Review of Philosophy*, *42*(2), 397–405.
Peña, C., & Silva, P. (Eds.) (2022). *Social Revolt in Chile: Triggering Factors and Possible Outcomes*. Routledge.
Proctor, H. (2024). *Burnout: The Emotional Experience of Political Defeat*. Verso.
Puar, J. (2017). *The Right to Maim: Debility, Capacity*. Duke University Press.
Richard, N. (2021). *Revuelta Social y Nueva Constitución*. CLACSO.
Ross, K. (2023). *The Politics and Poetics of Everyday Life*. Verso.
Wittgenstein, L. (2002). *Tractatus Logico-Philosophicus*. Routledge.

Žižek, S. (2008). *The Sublime Object of Ideology*. Verso.
Zupančič, A. (2024). *Disavowal*. Polity.

6
The Fantasy of Clairvoyance

Sociology is customarily taken as a proxy for the entire field of the social sciences—the former serving as shorthand for the latter, and vice versa (Susen, 2020). This privileged place in academia by no means derives from a clear consensus on sociology's role or even its object of enquiry. In fact, few debates are more recurrent within the discipline than that concerning the role of sociology itself. The frontrunners of each generation have all put forward their own definitions of sociology's task, yet there is little doubt that the discipline is seen as having a task to fulfil. From the second half of the twentieth century onwards, the sociological field in the West began to be more explicitly defined in terms of its critical or transformative potential (Keucheyan, 2013). In many ways, the first stone was thrown in 1937, when Max Horkheimer (2002) published his canonical essay 'Traditional and Critical Theory'. Written in response to what he deemed the pernicious consequences of sociology's professionalisation in capitalist societies, Horkheimer urged researchers to reject the prevailing modes of thought and to ground their practice 'not in the preservation of contemporary society but in its transformation into the right kind of society' (p. 218). It can be said that his call found receptive ears—so much so that, these days, it is non-critical sociology that appears

G. Sánchez, *A Rebel Unconscious*, Studies in the Psychosocial,
https://doi.org/10.1007/978-3-032-12275-9_6

in need of justification, rather than the other way around. Let me quote Luc Boltanski (2011, pp. 16–7) in extenso on this point:

> It remains the case that critique's dependence on sociology has as its corollary sociology's dependence on critique [...]. Who would be interested in a sociology for sociology's sake (in the way people refer to "art for art's sake") – that is to say, a sociology, which, exhausting itself in ever more sophisticated and meticulous descriptions, has no other objective than its own fulfilment as a discipline of knowledge? And furthermore, if it is accepted that this discipline can only have as its object the ways in which people, through their reflexive activity, make and break collectives, we can examine what the very content of this "knowledge" might be. The processes through which the actors in social life constitute the wholes of which they form part, and cause them to last or subvert them, are themselves articulated, in large measure, with the possibility of critique, not only when they challenge existing orders, but also when they are led to justify them. Sociology would be a strange activity if, out of a sort of misplaced modesty or sheepishness, it forbade itself a practice that contributes so significantly to the determination of its object. By dint of wishing to place the social world at a distance, as if in order to dominate it from without, it would deprive itself of what gives it a social foundation.

Boltanski stages a sort of hall of mirrors: sociology can only take as its object of enquiry the ways in which people make and break collectives, a process that is itself informed by critique. Social life is *directly* sociological or, which amounts to the same, *already* critical—hence, there is no reason for sociologists to succumb to modesty. This recalls the circular logic in Steven Buechler's (2008) essay 'What is Critical About Sociology', where he asserts that 'sociology is critical because thinking sociologically inevitably requires thinking critically' (p. 319). Even so, as he notes, the 'virtually universal support for critical thinking' (p. 318) might sit uneasily with the sociological community, insofar as it points to the hollowness of critique. We should ask ourselves why, after all, the acceptance of something deemed necessary would be considered problematic. The plot thickens further when we consider the vast literature on the erosion of critique in contemporary academia and the efforts required for its revival (e.g., Benson, 2021; Dörre et al., 2015; Fassin & Harcourt,

2019). This succinct overview suggests that we can, at once, argue that sociology and critique are one and the same, acknowledge that sociologists should be heedful of the contemporary extension of critique, and still recognise a perceived deficit in critical sociology. In the relationship between sociology and social change, there is a circle that proves remarkably difficult to square.

This chapter focuses on the tension outlined above. For reasons that will be fully developed later, in Latin America—and Chile in particular—sociologists have played not only an intellectual role in relation to the direction of social change, but also a practical one. According to one of the most thorough studies on the configuration of the sociological field in Latin America (Solari et al., 1976), the nature of sociology and the social role of sociologists were a concern from the very beginning. 'It is reasonable to suspect', the authors conclude, 'that, in relation to the total sociological production, nowhere in the developed or developing world has as much been written about this problem as in Latin America' (p. 62). Furthermore, for these authors, the standard divide between 'scientific' and 'critical' sociology is unfounded, as the latter seeks to expand the scope of science while assigning to the application of sociological knowledge a far more revolutionary potential. Consequently, the main focus of sociology in Latin America has been the region's defining problems—development, dependency, authoritarianism, democracy, and neoliberalism—and the ways in which sociological narratives might exert a performative role in shaping how these problems are addressed (see Garretón, 2007; Martuccelli & Svampa, 1993). While there is no general accord on how successfully sociologists have influenced the course of social affairs in Chile, the very fact that this debate is framed almost exclusively around the role of sociology (Ariztía, 2012; De Cea, 2018; Ramos, 2019) indicates that the discipline holds a position only rivalled by economics (Montecinos & Markoff, 2009) in shaping social change.

Despite coming from different disciplines, the weight of sociology is strongly felt in my interviewees' narratives—alongside the psychic tensions between expert knowledge about social change and the transformation of society already underway. My interpretation indicates that, contrary to how this debate is typically framed, the tension is not merely epistemological but also, and crucially, unconscious. Boltanski's hall of mirrors, in which sociology reflects the world and the world reflects sociology, is a motif present in nearly every critical sociological enterprise, yet its libidinal economy is rarely examined. The *estallido* embodies the psychic tensions of this deeply rooted belief: while the unfolding of social transformation in Chile may be seen as the triumph of sociology's critical impulse, it can simultaneously be experienced as a subjective loss. The imaginary assumption that the world we live in is, in some fundamental way, inherently sociological underpins this tension—precisely what the revolt called into question. Navigating this new landscape requires confronting the possibility that sociology may be less powerful than it imagined itself to be.

In Sociology More than Sociology

At the time of the interview, Carmen was a doctoral researcher. She has a strong background in sociology, complemented by further postgraduate training abroad. According to her own self-description, she is deeply committed to her discipline and an assiduous militant of one of the political parties in the coalition in power in Chile. As I have stated previously, I conducted all of my interviews in the same manner—I asked my interviewees if they can tell me the first thing that came to mind when I say *estallido social*, whatever that might be. For Carmen, the first thing that surfaced in her recollection was an anecdote from abroad with fellow compatriots.

> I remember, above all, a discussion I had with some [male Chilean] historians who told me: "How can it be that sociologists...?" – because I've worked in national and international research centres, you know? – and they told me: "How could it be that you didn't know this? How could it be that you didn't...?" As in, why I didn't almost get the exact date: "How could you not tell us that this shit was going to happen!?" Hmm, yeah. And I remember that, that, that relationship with other people who blamed us for not – and they blamed me in particular for being a militant – it was like: "You're a militant, you worked in those places, you did this and that, and you didn't know that this was going to happen!?" I don't know… I don't know if someone could have known-known – no

> one, no one. It surprises me today when people say things like: "But it was obvious!" I mean, yeah it was – somehow it was kinda obvious – but it wasn't; it's one of those loooong processes. Actually, I was just talking to a friend the other day who criticised the social sciences – she's a sociologist – and she said something like, she said exactly that: "How can it be that we didn't foresee this thing? How can it be that there are no good indicators to measure it, to anticipate these kinds of things?" And, I don't know man, I don't know – I don't know if the social sciences have that capacity, honestly.

Some background information is needed before attempting any interpretation of this rich excerpt. The international research centre she mentions has played an influential role in Chilean politics by furnishing decision-makers, academics, and politicians with interpretations of local socioeconomic trends. Since the mid-1990s, the centre's reports have explored the unintended consequences of Chile's modernisation path. According to an independent study, the reports have 'conspicuously embodied the function of public sociology' by adopting an interpretive standpoint that grants them a 'critical capacity' (Ramos, 2006, p. 126). Sociologists have historically occupied senior research positions within the teams responsible for these studies. The national research centre Carmen refers to, on the other hand, is one of the most prestigious social science hubs in the country. This is a multi-institutional endeavour with a focus on progressive social policy. It is divided into different areas and, as of 2025, half of them were led by sociologists.

Understanding the position that sociology occupies in Chilean academia, as well as in the political and cultural domains, is crucial to grasp what is at stake in Carmen's recollection. Different studies have shown the performative capacity of sociology in the country (Ariztía, 2012; De Cea, 2018; Ramos, 2012, 2019). Especially during the first decades after the end of the dictatorship, it has been said that sociologists 'contributed to the creation of the social in Chile by narrating the emerging society through general descriptions of change' (Ariztía & Bernasconi, 2012, p. 159). This role was enacted not only through academic research, but also via newly assumed advisory positions within the democratic governments. According to De Sierra et al. (2007), the post-dictatorship period in Latin America implied a rearrangement of the ties between social scientists and politics. A large number of the most qualified intellectuals, many of whom had taken part in the opposition to authoritarian regimes from exile, became political advisors or high-ranking public servants. The authors of the above study eloquently illustrate the magnitude of this reorganisation: 'The list of sociologists and political scientists who went on to serve in the governmental cadres of Chile, Argentina, and Brazil is as extensive as it is impossible to reproduce here' (De Sierra et al., 2007, p. 22). Thus, while the precise effects of sociology's performative capacity may be difficult to determine, there is ample evidence of sociologists' influence within the centre-left governments of Chile's post-dictatorship period. By way of example:

- Patricio Aylwin, the first democratically elected president after the dictatorship, appointed Ernesto Tironi, a renowned sociologist, as the government's head of communications.
- His successor, Eduardo Frei, named José Joaquín Brunner, a sociologist specialising in higher education, as a member of his cabinet.
- Ricardo Lagos, who came to power in 2000 under the promising banner of 'the first socialist president since Allende', introduced several governmental innovations. One of these was the creation of a permanent advisory team based at the presidential palace. Due to its location within the building, it was nicknamed 'the second floor'. During Lagos' presidency, this distinguished group of professionals was led by Ernesto Ottone, a senior sociologist trained in France.
- Michelle Bachelet, also a socialist, succeeded Lagos as the first woman ever elected president of Chile. She appointed Pedro Güell, an established sociologist, as the head of her second floor.
- The centre-left government of Gabriel Boric brought in Lucía Dammert, another sociologist whose field of expertise is international relations, to serve as director of his second floor.

The only interruption to this tradition of appointing sociologists to key government positions or senior advisory roles occurred during the presidency of Sebastián Piñera—the sole right-wing president of this period. As we have seen, both sociology and sociologists have been highly influential in the interpretation and conduct of Chilean affairs since 1990. Within the humanities and social sciences, their influence is rivalled only by that of economists.

With the above in mind, let me return to Carmen's experience. Her first association took the almost literal form of a confrontation with lack—Carmen was held accountable by her colleagues for sociology's failure to respond. Moreover, the makeup of the anecdote turns it into a scene akin to a trial: legal representatives of one discipline conducting an interrogation to return a verdict on whether Carmen, as the embodiment of sociology, has failed to deliver according to her remit. The questions directed at Carmen—'How could you not know?' and 'How could you not tell us?'—carry two implicit assumptions without which such demands for explanation would be meaningless: (1) you, as a sociologist, should have known; and (2) you, as a sociologist, should have informed us. Naturally, none of this took place; no one anticipated the *estallido*, and the very idea that someone ought to have known beforehand is patently unreasonable. This did not prevent those questions from being raised, and rather than responding dismissively, Carmen dwelt on them. This curious turn of events merits close exploration.

Many participants in my research expressed similar views about sociology. This was the case even though only two of them, Carmen and Sofía, were sociologists. Ramón, for example, qualified his statements on several occasions during our interviews with the adverb 'sociologically'. For him, there are many aspects of the revolt that are 'sociologically undeniable'—such as the violence and the growing perception of insecurity in recent years—while at the same time there are 'beautiful elements' of the *estallido* that lie 'beyond sociological analyses'. María, whose background is in education, addressed the various terms in circulation to name the *estallido*. After weighing the advantages and limitations of a few of them, she added: 'Because I'm not trained in sociology, I don't have like this need to consciously stand from such and such place; like to choose a word and take it as my, I don't know, my favourite word, and justify it'. When discussing academic publications on ongoing events, Verónica remarked that sociologists, unlike other scholars, 'are the ones who normally come up with books on these kinds of issues'. In a similar vein, Isabel shared her view that 'published academic explanations [of the *estallido*] weren't spot-on—I mean, the sociological explanations they gave were a little ridiculous sometimes'. Finally, Rodrigo's very first line in our interview was the following:

> The effects of the *estallido* were something that, in a way, people who study sociology, who are a bit aware of… I mean, you don't have to study sociology, because I tend to think that my reflections on the present come more from a political interest than from a disciplinary one, right? So, what one thinks about the *estallido* is that we were expecting it, in some way. I mean, it was not something that… it didn't take us by surprise.

In these vignettes, sociology emerges not so much as a discipline or field of enquiry, but as a guarantor of truth. To borrow Ramón's phrasing, sociology varnishes claims with a layer of undeniability. Owing to this function, it appears natural that sociologists are seen as those who select and justify the terms with which we name events—as well as those who produce and reproduce the collective literature surrounding them (even if, at times, they miss the mark). Rodrigo offers perhaps the most suggestive equivalence in this regard: people who study sociology = people who are aware of things. Immediately after drawing this correspondence, he corrects himself in a singular manner. At first glance, it seems he realises that it is not only those who study sociology who are attuned to the effects of the *estallido*. But instead of suggesting, for instance, that people who study other disciplines are just as aware, he reassured me that he works *in a manner similar to that of sociologists*. Ultimately, he makes himself part of the equivalence by 'sociologising' his own practice.

We should not overlook the fact that these associations represent a unique privilege granted to sociology alone. Sociology is not simply one discipline among others capable of making sense of the *estallido*—it is the only one. Or, as Isabel unwittingly suggested, academic explanations *are* sociological explanations. At no point in any of my interviews did a participant say something along the lines of 'historical analyses aside', 'anthropologically speaking', or 'avoiding psychological gestures' to frame their accounts. I held conversations with scholars representing almost the full gamut of the humanities and social sciences, yet only sociology appeared to possess this powerful capacity to render researchers immune to surprise—or at least to claim as much. Both what is said and what remains unsaid about other disciplines reveal an excessive, properly libidinal investment in sociology. In a sense, sociology goes beyond itself and becomes a fantasmatic site that delivers certitude—the extraordinary, and thoroughly unrealistic, capacity to turn radically contingent events into objects of foresight.

The Imaginary Grounds of Sociology

When we take sociology not as a discipline but as signifier that imaginarily mediates our relationship with expert knowledge in social change, things that initially appeared strange become more comprehensible. Historians can interpellate a sociologist on the basis of her lack of anticipatory knowledge because such a lack erodes the imaginary prowess of critical academia as a whole. The unconscious belief is that everyone can harbour doubt except sociologists—from within the coordinates of this fantasy, a surprised sociologist is a contradiction in terms. Carmen exhibits an ambivalent connection to this imaginary framework. She feels torn between the reasonable stance that 'no one could have known-known' the *estallido* would occur and the idea that it was 'kinda obvious'. In her speech, we can perceive a pendular movement, a sort of hesitation, between recognition and misrecognition within this oracular fantasy. The most pristine moment of misrecognition arises with the feeling of surprise at the generalised sense of obviousness permeating the people surrounding her. This is, nevertheless, a rather fleeting moment. She swiftly recoils from this feeling by suggesting that the emergence of the *estallido* was relatively obvious—a step that appears to move towards recognition. Later in our interview, while discussing the responsibility of the social sciences, Carmen articulates a moment of near-complete recognition with this imaginary side of sociology:

> [...] we [sociologists] are the only ones that, I think, the only ones that do have – at least in some respects – that do have the capacity, you know? Like, last year I was working very closely with lawyers, and lawyers fascinate me – I find them very interesting – because they just don't have...

> there are dimensions of social problems that they can't grasp, as simple as that, you know? But we [sociologists] do have the tools, so I often feel that those tools are there, but they are not used – out of convenience. Because fuck! with a paper on this or that topic, you know you'll definitely get published in X, Y, or Z journal, you know?

It seems difficult to find a clearer moment of identification with the association: people who study sociology = people who are aware of things. The misrecognition expressed through surprise, and the subsequent 'kinda obvious' hesitation, gives way here to an air of absolute certitude about the uniqueness of sociologists—they are the only ones with the capacity to comprehensively know things. This conviction is bolstered by—and indeed facilitated through—the lawyers, who occupy the discursive position of the other. The way she refers to them borders on the patronising: they fascinate her, she finds them very interesting because they are not as capable as sociologists, as simple as that. However, my claim is that this goes beyond merely disparaging former colleagues. The figure of the lawyer enables Carmen to secure her attachment to the imaginary possibilities that make sociology more than sociology.

Bearing in mind that a fantasy 'is the primordial form of *narrative*, which serves to occult some original deadlock' (Žižek, 1997, p. 11), we can perceive how the figure of the lawyer allows Carmen to entrench her attachment to sociology through a double movement. First, by way of comparison with a lacking other—who cannot grasp certain dimensions of social problems—sociology is able to retain the imaginary warrant of its purported predictive wholeness. Second, since sociologists in Carmen's account come dangerously close to occupying the same lacking position as the lawyers, the reason for not using their tools is externalised: these days, the conditions favour their abandonment. Owing to the incentives for publication and the ever-increasing pressure to keep doing so (Leyton & Sánchez, 2024; Macfarlane, 2021), sociological tools are misused. It seems that Carmen protects her attachment to sociology through the colonisation of bad knowledge over good knowledge: sociologists are the only ones who know-know things, but they also know how comfortable it is to get published. Sociologists have the tools, but they have grown too cosy within the university, so to speak—and that might be why they *seem* unable to anticipate what lies ahead.

The idea that sociology owns the tools, but sociologists were unable to use them properly during the *estallido*, also plays a significant role in Sofía's narrative. She is the other sociologist in my sample, and she shares both the political and professional commitments expressed by Carmen. 'I felt a bit frustrated', she admits, 'because this was a moment for sociology—and for what we could also contribute to it'. Frustration permeates many of her associations. Much like Carmen's view that the social sciences 'maybe weren't scratching where the itch was', Sofía's frustration stems from the conviction that, in the context of the radical demonstrations unfolding across the country, 'it was sociology's responsibility to rise to the challenge of its society'. In her view, that did not occur. Sofía draws on a well-known sociological concept to describe both what was happening on the streets and the source of her discipline's predicaments. For her, the *estallido* set in motion a process of generalised 'sociological imagination'. This terminology, rooted in the work of Charles Wright Mills (2000), allows her to suggest that Chileans were connecting their biographies with each another while simultaneously realising that the problems they were facing were structural in nature—and that they were making history.[1] Sofía glimpses a paradox here:

> So, the paradox I saw was that we were living through a moment when the discipline [sociology] was diminished. Diminished by the extreme specialisation, by the logic of productivity that values quantity over the capacity to influence society, and by a form of sociology that, at the same time, well, seemed to have no explanation for what was happening. So, I said: A moment of generalised sociological imagination is accompanied by a poor sociological imagination within the discipline. I mean, that's why we have to rise to the challenge, right? [...] I think many colleagues did have something to contribute in terms of explaining the moment – it's just that sociology is going through a crisis in its ability to influence the

[1] For further discussions connecting the *estallido* with the sociological imagination, see Canales and Duarte (2020) and Cortés (2019).

public. The spaces are dominated mainly by the technocrats' sociological imagination, and it's a very limited one.

Sofía and Carmen converge in attributing the lack of sociological explanations for the *estallido* to the same external condition—academic productivity. While Carmen emphasises how this dynamic encourages a more or less conformist disposition among sociologists, Sofía stresses that contemporary markers of academic success tend to curtail sociology's capacity for social impact. They are also aligned in their belief in sociology's ascendancy over other professions. The position occupied by lawyers in Carmen's account is taken by technocrats in Sofía's. Both groups acquire discursive value as representatives of lack, being mobilised essentially as not-sociologists or as bearers of un-sociological knowledge. Despite these similarities, Sofía's speech is nonetheless constructed around a distinctive set of associations that allow me to further delineate the fantasmatic dimension of sociology.

It would be fair to say that, alongside Durkheim's *The Rules of Sociological Method*, Weber's *The Methodology of the Social Sciences*, Bourdieu's *The Logic of Practice*, and a few others, Mills' *The Sociological Imagination* is one of the canonical works in the field when it comes to addressing what sociologists (should) do. Nearly every undergraduate sociology student is required to engage with it during their first year of training—myself included. Sofía's account, then, is firmly grounded in the sociological tradition.[2] My interest, however, is not in ascertaining how accurate her use of Mills' concept is, but rather in exploring the symbolic associations this notion enables. With only slight variation, the argument conveyed by Sofía in the excerpts above was also reiterated during the lessons I observed. In a session in late May 2022, for instance, she told her students that '[Chilean] society is kinda thinking in sociological terms, since the revolt enhanced the sociological imagination—but the social sciences are a bit stunned'. On the basis of this repetition, the

[2] The sociological imagination was also deployed to interpret the social unrest of 2011 in Chile. For Juan Pablo Rodríguez (2020), the social movements involved in this event renewed the power of social critique by situating individual problems within broader contexts. By creating new bonds of solidarity based on this connection, people 'create and carry out their own versions of Wright Mills' sociological imagination' (p. 8).

following question arises: could this rather technical term, sociological imagination, also reveal something about Sofía's unconscious desire for social change?

Imagination, in the context of the revolt, is not just a word among others. Many scholars and spokespersons for civil society organisations perceive that the *estallido* laid the groundwork for imagining Chile otherwise. It is against this backdrop that Sofía chose to draw on the heuristic tools provided by Mills. And one of the striking features of her account is the expansive reach the sociological imagination acquires in her speech. She repeatedly deployed the category to explain what, in her view, was unfolding as a result of the *estallido*. So, first of all, and contrary to her own conclusion, there was an explanation for what was happening—at least the one she offered via the sociological imagination. But if we look more closely at this explanation, it appears that the sociological imagination is used somewhat indiscriminately to name nearly any form of imagination. We hear about the publics' sociological imagination, the technocrats' sociological imagination, Chilean society's sociological imagination, and... the sociologists' sociological imagination—which, in turn, can be either good or poor. This marks a curious and voracious symbolic expansion for what is otherwise a strictly technical term—a feature that seems to express more than mere academic zeal.[3]

This extension of the sociological imagination bears a family resemblance to Carmen's claim that sociologists are the only ones capable of fully comprehending things. Here, under Sofía's discursive command, sociology becomes the yardstick by which imagination itself is measured; the quality of imagination is to be judged according to how sociological it is. On this basis, technocrats' imagination is deemed limited, as it is not sufficiently sociological. One might say that this entails a reification of an academic concept. In a way, it sounds as misplaced as claiming that technocrats' deconstructive tools are somewhat rusty. Expecting dexterity in the use of sociological—or, for that matter, philosophical—categories

[3] Mills addresses the adjective 'sociological' in his formulation in a singular fashion. In a footnote, he humorously recalls handing the manuscript of his book to colleagues from other social sciences, each of whom suggested adjectivising the imagination with their own discipline. 'The term matters less than the idea', Mills (2000, p. 19) reassuringly declares. If that is so, why not simply call it 'imagination'?

from technocrats, or indeed from any academic other than sociologists or philosophers, is plainly incongruous. But that is not the whole story. Sofía is not merely suggesting that other disciplines would benefit from incorporating sociological insights—which is actually a possible reading—but also, and ironically, that because others have adopted the sociological imagination, *sociologists themselves can no longer deploy it as they should*. This reveals that, for Sofía, the concept of 'sociological imagination' has an extra-theoretical or extra-epistemological value, insofar as it enables her to construct a fantasmatic scenario of wholeness.

Once again, in another May session, Sofía said: 'The social sciences are experiencing something quite strange [...]. What I'm saying is a tad contradictory, since what I'm saying is that there's a lack of sociological imagination and, also, that we did see the revolt coming'. My interpretation has tried to demonstrate that this is a *psychic contradiction.* Rather than a miscommunication between sociology and the public, what Carmen and Sofía were grappling with was the erosion of the recognition they found in the discipline's imaginary prophetic powers. In other words, the call of the Other of the *estallido* was incompatible with the possibility of having seen the revolt coming, as that would mean that social change never quite took place. Through different symbolic associations, Carmen and Sofía nonetheless express an equivalent libidinal attachment to transformative knowledge: insofar as sociologists are the only ones who know, and because they possess foretelling abilities, they must be heard.[4]

Based on my reading, what the *estallido* altered was not sociology's conceptual production, but the libidinal economy that organises its reproduction. If the whole point, according to Sofía, is to prop up 'a critical public sociology able to deliver the tools to address this kind of phenomenon', then there is no real problem since, by her own admission, Chilean society was already thinking in sociological terms as a result

[4] This bears an affinity to what Kristin Ross refers to as 'priestly sociology'. Following closely Jacques Rancière's attack on 'the Bourdieu effect'—that is to say, tautological sociological analysis—Ross (2023, p. 49) argues that, by virtue of this priestly stance, 'the sociologist places himself in the position of denouncing a system granted the ability to hide itself forever from its agents; the social critic sees what others cannot. His authority derives from the unknowingness of his objects of study'. It is worth noting that the Chilean sociological milieu has strong ties to its French counterpart, on account of postgraduate training and intellectual affinities.

of the revolt. In practical terms, there is no issue. At this precise point, however, we can discern how ambivalent her unconscious attachment truly is. While discussing the role played by the media during the revolt and how exhausting it was to counterbalance the overrepresentation of conservative political pundits, she suddenly perceives a silver lining. She does not regard this situation as overly problematic, since, during the *estallido*, the media 'gave a microphone to anyone, and that person made use of the sociological imagination that was happening'. Epistemologically, this is great news; the right tools for interpreting what was happening were within anyone's reach. Unconsciously, however, this was terrible news; the public was listening to *anyone*—not just sociologists, the rightful proprietors of those tools.

From this angle, Sofía's frustration takes on a new colouration. Despite the challenges of engaging in writing noted in the previous chapter, she constantly reproaches herself for not having done enough. 'Intellectually', Sofía admits, 'I wasn't doing all I could, because that basically meant writing down and recording everything—I mean, keeping a field notebook every day'. She then insists that she felt overwhelmed by her inability 'to do everything that needs to be done, to contribute everything that needs to be contributed. I felt limited—I couldn't do everything I wanted to do'. My take here is that, no matter how many pieces she might have written, this pressure to do everything would never have been assuaged since what is at stake is not the actual output of her work. This relentless eruption of the signifier 'everything' may be read as a response to the question Carmen was confronted with: 'How could you not tell us that this shit was going to happen!?', which is, in effect, another way of saying: You are a sociologist, why aren't you telling me the future? But, as Sofía admits, she now feels limited—unsuccessful in summoning a sense of wholeness.

I have been working on the basis that fantasies offer the subject a rationale for the inherent deadlock of desire. The experiences of both Carmen and Sofía show us that one of the primordial fantasmatic constructions is a scene 'in which the *jouissance* we are deprived of is concentrated in the Other who stole it from us' (Žižek, 1997, p. 43). Is this not precisely what Carmen and Sofía claim happened to them? At the very end of our conversation, Sofía solemnly said to me that 'the phase of being satisfied with what we've been saying is over', and subsequently closed our exchange by admitting that there are 'well-equipped' people within the sociological field to make a contribution, 'but what we lack is for any of this to affect reality, for someone to actually listen to what we're saying'. For Sofía, the 'right' tools had indeed been successfully passed onto the public; now *anyone* could use the sociological imagination. Unconsciously, however, this is experienced as a loss: sociology has no effect on reality because, for her, this seems to depend on a scenario in which *everyone* pays attention to what sociologists say. Put differently: now everybody is a clairvoyant, not just sociologists—which means that no one actually is. Summoning sociology, in this context, no longer produces the same effect. No matter how many pieces are put out there, without its imaginary grounds it becomes difficult to navigate the misrecognition of the Other. The concept of sociological imagination can, of course, still be deployed—it can even be serviceable—yet its libidinal economy has ceased to offer the coherence it once did.

Sociology's Imperial Unconscious

Public sociology, the most recent endeavour to reinvigorate critique within the sociological field, is profoundly indebted to Mills' sociological imagination. Michael Burawoy, its chief proponent and ardent defender, not only framed his *Public Sociology* (2021) as a means of renewing the 'promise' of sociology—paying homage to Mills' characterisation of the discipline and the purpose of its imagination—but even wrote letters addressed to him (Burawoy, 2008). In this public display of sociological affection, Burawoy spares no effort in expressing how much the present generation of sociologists owes to Mills' work: 'The notion that the sociological imagination is a quality of mind that turns personal troubles into public issues is perhaps the most oft-repeated mantra of the sociologist's self-representation' (p. 368). This overt admiration, however, is interspersed with some criticism. In Burawoy's view, if Mills was right in advancing the sociological imagination as the quintessential procedure for social analysis, he nevertheless went too far in his diatribe against professional sociology. What Mills failed to recognise was their mutual interdependence: without professional sociology, public sociology risks devolving into mere moral critique; without public sociology, professional sociology risks hardening into technocratic administration. For Burawoy, Mills succeeded in giving sociology a radical hue, but his animosity towards professional sociology prevented him from appreciating all its shades.

What is so radical about the sociological imagination? Like many sociologists before and after him, Mills diagnosed his era as being characterised by profound and accelerating transformations that were not effectively accompanied by the cognitive capacities needed to render them intelligible. For him, what people require is not better sociological interpretations, but rather 'a quality of mind that will help them to use information and to develop reason in order to achieve lucid summations of what is going on in the world and of what may be happening within themselves' (Mills, 2000, p. 5). This quality of mind is the sociological imagination. In a nutshell, it refers to the capacity to bridge interpretive scales within a single analytic procedure—to perceive how history intersects with biography and to grasp their mutual implications within society. For Mills, this capacity is both a task and a promise: something that must be undertaken and kept alive. Such a quality of mind carries deep emancipatory potential, resonant with the Chilean revolt:

> The sociological imagination is the most fruitful form of this self-consciousness. By its use men whose mentalities have swept only a series of limited orbits often come to feel *as if suddenly awakened* in a house with which they had only supposed themselves to be familiar. (Mills, 2000, pp. 7–8, emphasis added)

Some researchers have noted that this quality of mind, which has become central to sociologists' self-representation in Burawoy's view, harbours a problematic side. For Thomas Kemple and Renisa Mawani (2009), the sociological imagination casts an imperial shadow over the social sciences. What Mills' device effectively does is to turn a specific model of knowledge production into the default epistemological standard, making the American style of sociology a one-size-fits-all solution to any concern about social life. As Andrew Sayer (1999, p. 2) shrewdly observes in his reflections on disciplinary imperialism, extending a discipline's territorial claims is most commonly achieved by 'shifting from grounding themselves in a topic or object of study to identifying themselves in terms of ways of seeing'. The sociological imagination performs precisely this move: more than a *sociological* method, it becomes a *universal* quality of mind. As per Kemple and Mawani, it is hard not to see the parallels between the sociological imagination and the imperial drive of the United States. In this sense, despite the sociological attention given to the study of imperialism, such literature has not substantially altered the ways in which the discipline's 'ontological moorings, categories, and modes of analysis have been fundamentally structured by imperial pursuits and formed within cultures of colonialism' (Kemple & Mawani, 2009, p. 238). This is why, for them, the sociological imagination enacts its own version of this 'imperial unconscious'.

This line of thought draws inspiration from Raewyn Connell's (1997) reassessment of the sociological canon. Taking as her starting point what she identifies as two key anomalies of sociology's classics—first, that despite their alleged prestige, much social research simply ignores them in practice; and second, that the canonical authors themselves did not embrace the origin story the canon would later cement—she seeks to uncover the historical function of the canon. To simplify her otherwise highly scrupulous argument, she contends that the emergence of the sociological canon should be understood not through internalist models but in geopolitical terms. In other words, the time and place in which the canon materialised is the decisive factor: 'Sociology was formed within the culture of imperialism and embodied a cultural response to the colonized world. This fact is crucial in understanding the content and method of sociology as well as the discipline's cultural significance' (Connell, 1997, p. 1519). Sociology's comparative method, then, was less a response to an internal or epistemological need than an expression of the imperial gaze of the period (see also Go, 2013a; Steinmetz, 2013).

Alongside Kemple and Mawani, Julian Go (2013b) and Steven Seidman (2013) also refer to this feature of sociology in terms of the 'imperial unconscious' and the 'colonial unconscious', respectively. Their investigations further develop Connell's geopolitical argument by demonstrating the various avenues through which sociology has reproduced an imperial epistemology: 'In short, American sociology shifted away from its imperial and global framework as the twentieth century proceeded. But its new modes of theory and research still carried the traces of a lingering and deep-rooted imperial unconscious' (Go, 2013b, p. 104). In all these analyses, 'unconscious' is used as an adjective to describe an attribute of sociology, taking on a metaphorical tone. Unconscious becomes synonymous here with unintended, silent, or hidden. After the political disintegration of empires, some of their logics survived in epistemological form, *unwittingly* informing sociological practice. In these accounts—even in Connell's radical reappraisal of sociological theory—sociology's potency is never in question. The discipline may have an unglamorous origin and may have partaken in some reproachable enterprises, but these are treated as unintended attributes. So much so that, as the preceding studies demonstrate, sociology can redeem itself by examining its own 'hidden' traits.

My interpretation of the experiences of Carmen and Sofía points not to a metaphorical but rather to a very literal sense of sociology's imperial unconscious. To say it directly: the call of the Other of the revolt is experienced as a loss because, for them, *the world is no longer coterminous with sociology*. The imaginary ground of the sociological imagination is the idea that the world and the discipline are one and the same. The sociological imagination can be presented as *the* quality of mind required to make sense of the world because, for sociology, the world is already composed of sociological particles. Given this assumption, it becomes only natural to evaluate others' mental capacities in relation to the sociological imagination—ultimately, there is no other imagination imaginable. This imaginary position entails at least two structural contradictions. First, if sociology and the world are indeed coextensive, then sociologists should not need to exhaust themselves trying to convince us of something already inscribed in the fabric of reality. The fact that they do implies that this coextensiveness is, to a large extent, an effect produced by the very efforts to demonstrate its obviousness. Second, even if every interpretation could be considered an instance of the sociological imagination, it is still sociologists who are deemed the ones entitled to deploy it.

Both contradictions came to light during the revolt, throwing a spanner in the imaginary works of Carmen and Sofía. When Sofía observes that the Chilean people were making use of the tools of public sociology and the sociological imagination, she cannot help but experience this as a loss: if *anyone* can wield the sociological tools during the revolt, then her foretelling powers are no longer being heeded—even though, against all odds, *sociologists* did in fact see the revolt coming. This is the moment when she is confronted with the possibility that the fabric of the world may not be intrinsically sociological after all. A similar rupture occurred for Carmen when she was held accountable by colleagues for not having predicted the *estallido*—a moment when sociological capacity itself is perceived as faltering. And what is the response to this? To frame it as an external opposition of forces rather than as the consequence of an internal contradiction. External mechanisms such as academic capitalism, performance culture, or the media are blamed for preventing sociologists from acknowledging that they had foreseen the revolt. This manoeuvre serves to fend off a more unsettling possibility, namely, that the world is no longer an imaginary extension of themselves. As Alberto Toscano (2012, p. 72) puts it, 'the Millsian desire to see it whole' proves here to be, very literally, an unconscious desire.

The interpretation I have offered in this chapter suggests that critical sociology rests on imaginary assumptions that make the experience of social change hard to endure for social scientists. The main assumption, pristinely conveyed by the sociological imagination, is the idea that the world is composed of a sociological substance. This places sociology in the position of *primus inter pares* within the social sciences, a status that is both internally assumed and externally recognised. The belief that sociology and the world are coextensive gives rise to an imperial unconscious, which manifests in a sense of wholeness that cannot tolerate alienation—from within sociology's jurisdiction, there is no room for lack. Sociologists are the only ones who know, the ones who can see things coming, because they are one with the world. And yet, at the same time, they must also *conquer that world*—as Sofía puts it, the revolt 'was a moment *for sociology*'. The experiences of Carmen and Sofía reveal the unconscious side of this contradiction, along with the imaginary mechanisms through which they sought to push alienation away.

During the revolt, they felt frustrated that sociology proved incapable of doing *more*: amid the conscious celebration of the world's transformation, their unconscious desire was to preserve the equivalence between sociology and the world. In this sense, Carmen and Sofía embodied the psychic tensions of critical sociology. This is precisely what contemporary efforts to bring the discipline closer to the public tend to gloss over: that 'public sociology is produced by publics even before they encounter professional sociologists' (Meghji, 2024, p. 122). To aspire to change the world while reinforcing its imaginary equivalence with sociology comes at a heavy psychic cost.

In *Sociology in the Twenty-First Century: Key Trends, Debates, and Challenges*, Simon Susen (2020) inadvertently provides the most graphic example of the imaginary grounds of sociology explored in this chapter. Intended as a way of illustrating the fragmentation of the discipline, Susen inventories 119 sociological subfields—the list spans four pages. Among them, we find 'critical sociology' (in the first position), 'sociology of critique', 'sociology of nothing', and even 'etc.' (pp. 264–267). The last two additions are key: in case sociologists have not yet discovered all the ways in which the world is already sociological, rest assured they will; and if something is not in the world, it might as well be sociological. A real transformation of the world such as that brought about by the *estallido* proves that the world is not coextensive with sociology—this is what Carmen and Sofía, as well as those around them, were at psychic pains to confront. Their commitment to social change is in no way bogus, but rests on a libidinal economy that demands control, predictability, and the supernatural capacity to know things in advance. Sayer (1999, p. 5) maintains that 'to know how far sociological explanations can be taken, we have to decide how far things cannot be explained sociologically'. Incapable of deciding this, Carmen and Sofía unconsciously experienced social change largely as a loss. Much like in Mills' description quoted above, they came to feel as if suddenly awakened in a house with which they had only supposed themselves to be familiar. But the fantasmatic certainty of the sociological imagination was no longer in place to make the unfamiliar familiar again. The revolt was properly uncanny for them.

References

Ariztía, T. (Ed.). (2012). *Produciendo lo Social*. Ediciones Universidad Diego Portales.

Benson, D. (Ed.). (2021). *Domination and Emancipation: Remaking Critique*. Rowman & Littlefield.

Boltanski, L. (2011). *On Critique: A Sociology of Emancipation*. Polity.

Buechler, S. (2008). What Is Critical About Sociology? *Teaching Sociology, 36*(4), 318–330.

Burawoy, M. (2008). Open Letter to C. *Wright Mills. Antipode, 40*(3), 365–375.

Burawoy, M. (2021). *Public Sociology: Between Utopia and Anti-Utopia*. Polity.

Canales, M., & Duarte, K. (2020). Imaginación sociológica para estudiar juventudes. *Última Década, 54*, 216–227.

Connell, R. (1997). Why Is Classical Theory Classical? *American Journal of Sociology, 102*(6), 1511–1557.

Cortés, A. (2019). La rebelión social como imaginación sociológica colectiva. *Cuadernos De Teoría Social, 5*(10), 77–93.

De Cea, M. (2018). The Role of Public Sociology in the Development of Cultural Policies in Chile: A Transformation of Cultural Expertise. *International Journal of Politics, Culture, and Society, 31*(2), 145–159.

De Sierra, G., Garretón, M., Murmis, M., & Trindade, H. (2007). Las ciencias sociales en América Latina en una mirada comparativa. In H. Trindade (Coord.), *Las Ciencias Sociales en América Latina en Perspectiva Comparada*. Siglo Veintiuno Editores.

Dörre, K., Lessenich, S., & Rosa, H. (2015). *Sociology, Capitalism, Critique*. Verso.

Fassin, D., & Harcourt, B. (Eds.) (2019). *A Time for Critique*. Columbia University Press.

Garretón, M. (2007). Las ciencias sociales en Chile. Institucionalización, ruptura y renacimiento. In H. Trindade (Coord.), *Las Ciencias Sociales en América Latina en Perspectiva Comparada*. Siglo Veintiuno Editores.

Go, J. (Ed.) (2013a). *Postcolonial Sociology*. Emerald.

Go, J. (2013b). Sociology's imperial unconscious: The Emergence of American Sociology in the Context of Empire. In G. Steinmetz (Ed.), *Sociology and Empire: The Imperial Entanglements of a Discipline*. Duke University Press.

Horkheimer, M. (2002). Traditional and Critical Theory. In *Critical Theory: Selected Essays*. Continuum.

Kemple, T., & Mawani, R. (2009). The Sociological Imagination and Its Imperial Shadows. *Theory, Culture & Society, 26*(7–8), 228–249.

Keucheyan, R. (2013). *The Left Hemisphere*. Verso.

Leyton, D., & Sánchez, G. (2024). Beyond (and alongside) Shameful Attachments: The Lived Experience of Critique Within the Entrepreneurial University. *Cultural Studies ↔ Critical Methodologies, 24*(4), 251–262.

Macfarlane, B. (2021). The Neoliberal Academic: Illustrating Shifting Academic Norms in an Age of Hyper-Performativity. *Educational Philosophy and Theory, 53*(5), 459–468.

Martuccelli, D., & Svampa, M. (1993). Notas para una historia de la sociología en Latinoamérica. *Sociológica, 8*, 23.

Meghji, A. (2024). From Public Sociology to Sociological Publics: The Importance of Reverse Tutelage to Social Theory. *Sociological Theory, 42*(2), 114–136.

Montecinos, V., & Markoff, J. (Eds.). (2009). *Economists in the Americas*. Edward Elgar.

Ramos, C. (Coord.) (2006). *El Impacto de los Informes de Desarrollo Humano del PNUD en Chile*. Departamento de Sociología de la Universidad Alberto Hurtado.

Ramos, C. (2012). *El Ensamblaje de Ciencia Social y Sociedad*. Ediciones Universidad Alberto Hurtado.

Ramos, C. (2019). *Relatos Sociológicos y sociedad. Tomás Moulian, José Joaquín Brunner y Pedro Morandé: Obra, Redes de Producción y Efectos (1965–2018)*. Ediciones Universidad Alberto Hurtado.

Rodríguez, J. P. (2020). *Resisting Neoliberal Capitalism in Chile: The Possibility of Social Critique*. Palgrave Macmillan.

Ross, K. (2023). *The Politics and Poetics of Everyday Life*. Verso.

Sayer, A. (1999). Long live postdisciplinary studies! Sociology and the curse of disciplinary parochialism/imperialism. Department of Sociology, Lancaster University.

Seidman, S. (2013). The Colonial Unconscious of Classical Sociology. In J. Go (Ed.), *Postcolonial Sociology*. Emerald.

Solari, A., Franco, R., & Jutkowitz, J. (1976). *Teoría, Acción Social y Desarrollo en América Latina*. Siglo Veintiuno Editores.

Steinmetz, G. (Ed.). (2013). *Sociology and Empire: The Imperial Entanglements of a Discipline*. Duke University Press.

Susen, S. (2020). *Sociology in the Twenty-First Century: Key Trends, Debates, and Challenges*. Palgrave Macmillan.

Toscano, A. (2012). Seeing it Whole: Staging Totality in Social Theory and Art. *The Sociological Review, 60*(1), 64–83.
Mills, C. W. (2000). *The Sociological Imagination.* Oxford University Press.
Žižek, S. (1997). *The Plague of Fantasies.* Verso.

7

The Fantasy of Powerlessness

Michel Foucault (2010) conceptualised neoliberalism as a historical shift in the way liberal societies produce individuals. His brilliance lay in identifying emerging mechanisms of political power aimed at shaping individuals who would mirror 'not the man of exchange, the consumer or the producer, but the enterprise' by inducing behaviours aligned with 'competition in terms of plans and projects, and with objectives, tactics, and so forth' (p. 175). These embryonic mechanisms of political power, which marked a departure from classical liberal ideas, have since developed considerably, turning Foucault's governmental perspective into the dominant framework for analysing the neoliberalisation of the world (Bevir, 2016; Lemm & Vatter, 2014; Rose, 1996). Against this backdrop, few domains have attracted more interest than education in efforts to understand the intricate plans, projects, objectives, and tactics whereby competition is activated to govern individuals (Ball, 2010, 2013; Besley & Peters, 2007). Among the reasons for this attention is the rise of the knowledge economy, which has turned the university into a pillar of the global market, reducing its public status and reorienting it towards profit-making and investment (Peters & Jandrić, 2018). The

G. Sánchez, *A Rebel Unconscious*, Studies in the Psychosocial,
https://doi.org/10.1007/978-3-032-12275-9_7

university has thus become a privileged site for analysing the manifold neoliberal strategies to regulate conduct through competition.

One of the consequences of shaping individuals to conform to the logic of the enterprise is that the latter ceases to function merely as an economic device and instead becomes a cultural logic (Marttila, 2018). This shift has produced conflicting dynamics within the university. At an organisational level, scholars have documented the replacement of public good models of governance with managerial forms of regulation that place emphasis on incentives, performance, and accountability (Leyton, 2022; Olssen, 2016). In the name of innovation and creativity, such mechanisms have entrenched managerial authority within the university, granting it the power not only to allocate resources but, by the same token, to define the academic mission itself (Newfield, 2019). For academics, the neoliberal elevation of managerial authority has transformed the principle of professional autonomy in matters of teaching and research. This has led to claims of an ongoing de-professionalisation of academic staff (Olssen & Peters, 2005), who have witnessed the steady erosion of their rights and control over their work. Ironically, one outcome of the infusion of managerial innovation and creativity is an intensification of pressure on what is researched, resulting in the stifling of researchers' creativity (Olssen, 2016). Accordingly:

> The literature describes how neo-liberal economic policies in higher education have resulted in the deterioration of working conditions and a loss of power by academic staff, manifested as managerialism, reduced funding, massification, external accountability, performativity, growing job insecurity, increased class sizes and growing accountability requirements, resulting in increased stress and work overload. (Kenny, 2018, pp. 377–378)

This chapter grapples with the loss of power experienced by academics. In Chile, research shows that managerial techniques used to control academic labour have a distinctive relationship with critique. For example, in the social sciences, a commitment to social change is mobilised in scholars' self-descriptions as a way of countering the pressure of performance metrics (Fardella, Sisto & Jiménez, 2015; Leyton &

Sánchez, 2024). Amid constant applications for research grants, submissions to high-impact journals, and the individualisation of academic work, a sense of responsibility to strive for social change through research emerges from academics' narratives. While this can certainly be perceived as a form of resistance to academic capitalism, it may also reinforce the productivist mandate by galvanising a sacrificial disposition to never stop. In many respects, the *estallido* released this commitment to social change from its managerial constraints. In the wake of the popular uprising, academics sought to contribute to the understanding of unfolding events through modes of intervention that managerial creativity would ordinarily suppress—interventions that were exploratory, collaborative, and unconcerned with metrics (e.g., Araujo, 2019; Balbontín & Salas, 2020; Henríquez & Pleyers, 2023).

In spite of the above, my interviews also show how the revolt neatly fitted into competitive research funding schemes, one of the quintessential managerial mechanisms of the modern university. As many academics declared, the *estallido* was annexed to their existing research grants or became a platform for securing new ones. The default explanation in the literature is that this reflects the incomplete nature of managerial capture over academic life: the neoliberal project is not coherent but rather properly 'mutant' (Callison & Manfredi, 2019), meaning that everyday neoliberalism in academia is navigated through 'tactical evaluations' that respond to the 'mismatch between the values of academic communities and capitalistic imperatives' (Cannizzo, 2018, p. 89). In a word, academics resemble a pendulum: their loss of power in the face of managerial control leads them to oscillate between compliance and resistance. From this perspective, the *estallido* informed both positions: it was an event that enabled scholars to resist the managerial grip by exercising creative modes of research, while also offering an opportunity to subsume it within performance evaluation.

I take an alternative route to explore this. The diminishing of academics' power since the inception of neoliberal modernisation is undeniable, particularly in places like Chile, where this this process was implemented by a dictatorship with the explicit aim of depoliticising the university (Rifo, 2017). But psychoanalysis demonstrates that two things can be true at once: 'we have already found often enough that in psychoanalysis opposites imply no contradiction' (Freud, 1991, p. 342). Just as Chapter 5 showed that impotence can have a counterintuitive psychic allure in the midst of the revolt, here I explore the psychic life of academics' loss of organisational and agential power, which can give rise to unexpected unconscious gains. When talking about the *estallido*, academics openly referred to their competitive research grants as if these created a space outside the sphere of power—an imaginary separation sustained by their own sense of exclusion from that very power. In their accounts, the world is not simply divided between the haves and the have-nots, but also includes an imaginary *having in order not to have*. Powerlessness may well be the result of four decades of managerial administration of the university, yet nothing prevents it from also functioning as an unconscious mechanism for managing this very lack of power.

John Clarke (2017) proposes approaching the neoliberal modernisation of the university in the terms delineated above. He suggests that the contradictory nature of this transformation may give rise to the emergence of 'collective psychic states', where this contradiction can be accommodated. 'The modernised university', Clarke maintains, 'is a powerful site of *fantasy*' (p. 142). This includes not only managerial fantasies of building a 'world-class' university, but also what he describes as 'dissociative' states that organise the everyday life of academic staff. He notes that, in response to the pervasiveness of leadership styles aimed at inspiring academic workers, some may withdraw into 'forms of privatised retreatism (the desire to be "left alone" with one's work)' (p. 143). A similar impulse emerged in my interviews. However, I suspect that what I encountered is not merely dissociative. In the context of what is widely seen as the most empowering event in recent Chilean history, academics appear uncertain about what to do with power—relying instead on imaginary constructions of powerlessness. Their approach to academic research, therefore, reveals a great deal about their unconscious identification with social change.

All Academic Roads Lead to *Fondecyt*

Until the revolt's momentum was suddenly interrupted by the pandemic in March 2020, the prevailing impression was that Chile had become an entirely different country. For the most part, this also applied to the university as well. Most universities remained closed for several months, and some restructured their regular activities to help make sense of the ongoing situation. Isabel's experience, for instance, is that 'the university came to a standstill, and everything was refocused on the revolt; research topics were reconfigured and, for instance, I asked my students to engage with the *estallido* in their final essays'. Similarly, for Ramón the transformation was so profound that 'labour relations changed, universities changed, classrooms changed; I don't know – everything was turned upside down, everything was turned upside down'. This was unequivocally the case, although not the whole picture. Life within the university was far less monolithic and more nuanced than such wholesale reshaping suggests. Daniela's experience, for instance, shares some commonalities but diverges significantly from this account. As a 'taxi lecturer'—the local slang for a part-time scholar working across several institutions—she divided her time between her doctoral training and her teaching positions at two higher education institutions. What follows is her account of her working life while the revolt was unfolding:

> I was working at this very neoliberal private university at that time and, I don't know, I remember we were in a room with the students, and the day before a lot of people had lost their eyes [because of police brutality]. And the head of department was very clear: we weren't allowed to say anything. I mean, you had to teach your lessons, just carry on as if nothing was happening. [...] But I was also working at a public university, in a research centre, and it was really interesting because we held some political meetings there – it was something completely different. I kinda lived both sides; it was very schizophrenic.

Daniela found herself torn between an institutional directive to carry on with business as usual from her private employer and a more empathic and reflective response from her public one. This was not only her personal experience but, more broadly, a fair depiction of the general response of Chilean universities. By way of example, the largest public institution in the country, the University of Chile, became heavily engaged with the course of events. The institution facilitated multiple discussion forums and sponsored both academic and non-specialist publications, while its Vice-Chancellor openly expressed support for several popular demands arising from the revolt. And although it would be inaccurate to claim that this was exclusively the approach of public universities, similar initiatives from private institutions appear, to a large extent, to have depended on individual rather than organisational commitment. Consequently, and notwithstanding some exceptions, the *estallido* laid bare the differences between public and private institutions in their approaches to political change.

Academic research and publication form a domain that, regardless of the institutional nature, remained firmly in place during and after the *estallido*. In Chile, many of the publications are the result of funding granted to scholars by the National Agency for Research and Development. Between 1980 and 1981, the dictatorship carried out a sweeping transformation of higher education adducing as evidence the system's irrational and inorganic growth, its monopolistic nature and lack of proper regulation, and the socially regressive character of free tertiary education (Rifo, 2017). The neoliberal ethos of the 1981 reform introduced 'a set of new dynamics of institutional differentiation, diversification of educational provision, innovation opportunities for education entrepreneurs, and new funding mechanisms for higher education' (Brunner, 2015, p. 42). Among these mechanisms, that same year saw the establishment of the National Fund for Scientific and Technological Development (*fondecyt*, by its Spanish acronym). This public programme became the first competitive funding scheme introduced by the Chilean government as part of a broader policy shift in the allocation of public resources for higher education and scientific research. To this day, *fondecyts* remain not only the chief source of research funding, but also a central marker of academic prestige in Chile.

Perhaps the clearest indication of how deeply the logic of *fondecyt* has shaped the research landscape in Chile comes from one of my classroom observations. In early May 2022, I was granted access to

Verónica's module. That day, the lesson revolved around Charles Fourier's Harmony, the name he gave to his utopian world. The pleasure-seeking society he proposes is founded on a thorough reorganisation of social interactions, governed by new laws of passionate attraction. In his utopia, passions are not to be repressed but properly channelled. To achieve such an outcome, Fourier aspired to create mathematical equations for the calculation of passions, as well as a centralised information system of personal data. In keeping with these principles, he exhibited a penchant for assigning numbers to everything. When the importance attributed to food in Harmony was discussed during the lesson—Fourier, for instance, abhorred bread because it represented necessity rather than desire—Verónica mentioned that he had devised a list of nine dishes for his utopian setting. This prompted the joke from one of the students that made several others beam in complicity: 'That REALLY is a *fondecyt*!' This innocent piece of banter nevertheless reveals that even within a utopian world, a *fondecyt*-less research life seems unthinkable in Chile.

Some researchers, of course, are keenly aware, and at times vocally critical, of the perils of *fondecyt*. Carlos and Rodrigo, for instance, are among its most adamant opponents. Carlos argues that by enshrining publishing in high-impact, English language journals as both the selection criterion for funding and the desired outcome of funded projects, emerging topics—such as the *estallido*—are often incorporated into existing research agendas in an inorganic fashion. In other words, due to the imperative to maximise research products, urgent issues tend to be assimilated rather than genuinely explored. Rodrigo, in turn, highlights the flipside of Carlos' argument: that by adhering to *fondecyt*'s requirements, no phenomenon remains beyond academic reach; however, this very incorporation places such phenomena within a neoliberal economy of knowledge. Unless one is an exceptionally depoliticised scholar, this is a well-worn argument in Chile. Yet Rima Majed's (2023, p. 80) caveat, that 'revolutionary moments are often imbued with contradictory features and dynamics', seems particularly apt here, since both of Carlos and Rodrigo held *fondecyt* projects at the time of our interviews. And this is far from an isolated case. Verónica, too, embodies a similar contradiction:

> So, the revolt hit from every front: teaching, research, and my work as... because deep down, it was like – like a kind of conviction to act in a revolutionary way, let's say, wherever one happened to be. Yeah, that was it: a disruption in the existing order of things. [...] And that happened to many of us – we talk about it a lot, like: "So, how do I make the revolution here, here, and here?"

As Verónica maintains, her commitment to the *estallido* as a revolution is unshakable. For her, the radius of the *estallido*'s explosion encompassed every aspect of academic life, meaning that, in her own words, teaching and research must also become sites where the revolution is made. During the first and most effervescent weeks of the revolt, Verónica's new book arrived from the publishing house that had commissioned it. The book was part of a larger *fondecyt* project. She recalls taking part in a demonstration around Dignity Square carrying a handful of copies of her new book while asking herself: '"What do I even do with this thing in the *estallido*?" I mean, research-wise, what's the point of launching a book when everything's shut down?' The question she posed to herself is a layered one. She was, of course, pointing to how counterproductive it seemed to launch a scholarly book at a time when academic life, as we know it, is nowhere to be found: universities were closed and this undoubtedly felt like a poor timing for customary academic activities. Yet rhetorically asking, 'What do I do with this thing *in the estallido*?' also seems to imply an incompatibility between the book and the revolt.

I suggest reading Verónica's question in conjunction with her commitment to revolutionising all aspects of life. When considered together, her question is no longer merely rhetorical or illustrative of the irony of receiving a book when academic activities are suspended. In the midst of an event demanding one 'make the revolution here, here, and here', Verónica received the finished product of an unrevolutionised—or, at best, yet-to-be-revolutionised—research logic: her *fondecyt*. The perceived incompatibility, then, does not stem from the content of the book itself, but from what it represents in the context of the *estallido*. Yet the very *fondecyt* project from which her book emerged also enabled Verónica to publish articles on the revolt. This was possible, she explains, because the revolt 'didn't deviate my work too much', so 'I framed my text on the *estallido* there [in my *fondecyt*]; it fitted there'. What seems to surface in Veronica's account is the tension between the revolutionary character of the revolt and the stabilising logic of competitive research funding—*fondecyt*'s capacity to keep things in their usual place even amid radical social change.

A similar tension runs through Isabel's account. Although she does not see eye to eye on the idea of revolution, she nevertheless agrees that the *estallido* transformed both the country and the university at their core. In her view, the revolt gave rise to several forms of academic activism. People from law schools were advising and representing demonstrators in legal cases; medical faculty were providing aid on the streets; and scholars from social work departments were documenting police abuses and human rights violations. Like many other academics, she devoted a considerable amount of time and energy to such tasks, lending a hand where needed. Towards the end of our interview, she even remarked that, in her circles, many scholars have stepped away from the university—or seriously considered doing so—because this wave of academic activism made the extractivist nature of academic labour more visible than ever. Despite this awareness, she openly acknowledged that, alongside other colleagues, 'we were in the middle of a *fondecyt* on memory, the dictatorship, the post-dictatorship, and the transition, so what happened [with the *estallido*] fitted our research like a glove (laughs)'. Somehow, Isabel managed to get the best of both worlds: 'Cos being out there and seeing all that politicisation also helped my current *fondecyt* project, you know?' The articles she wrote on the *estallido* stand as evidence that this was indeed the case.

A Matter of Pins

How should we interpret the contradiction expressed above? How can the revolt fit so neatly into competitive funding schemes that run counter to the experience of the end of neoliberalism? I believe we would miss the point if we simply endorsed the idea that this is nothing but cynicism—even if cynicism might play a role in it. A different avenue to explore would be to interpret the fantasmatic role that *fondecyts* can perform *vis-à-vis* perceptions of the university, the place where these projects are carried out. And this is the case because, with varying degrees of animosity, virtually all the participants in my study expressed negative views of the university. 'One doesn't trust universities', is a laconic remark that came out of Carlos' mouth but could easily have been uttered by any of my interviewees. So much so, in fact, that both he and Ramón referred to the university as 'mafias'. Ramon's speech is so rich in this respect that it is worth quoting at length:

> I'm interested in an academic career in the sense of being able to do what I enjoy – winning research grants and supervising doctoral students, that's what I like. But that's where I draw the line; I'm not interested in a position, I'm not interested in the deanship, I'm not interested in anything that comes from an institution like the university. Because every time I get involved in something like accreditation and all that shit, I come out wanting to vomit. I mean, I find it absolutely disgusting [...]. And I think it's a mafia: two peers, who get paid, come in, and then these guys, I don't know... we all just say everything's great, and they hand out however many years [of accreditation] they're going to hand out. So yeah, it's kind of a mafia, man – this is what mafias do. Mafias do that kind of thing. Like Corleone, man: you're taking over more territory. It's just a matter of having more pins [*chapas*] or fewer pins, that's all.

The process he is describing, higher education accreditation, is a highly criticised one in Chile, owing to the lack of transparency and accountability of quality assurance agencies. Whether their methods resemble those of a mafia is open to debate. What piques my curiosity is the striking contradiction that arises when an academic declares disinterest in anything that comes from the university. Given that the job he chose, the identity he has forged, and the joy he derives from research all depend on the university, he must, at the very least, have some interest in such an institution. Yet he adamantly insists otherwise. Where does this need to discursively distance himself from an institution with which he is so evidently entangled come from? One possible answer is that, for him, the university is synonymous with a brawl for power. Somehow, he pulls off a subtle opposition: research is separated from the 'positions' available at the university, despite the fact that all of these activities take place within the same institutional setting. Put differently, what he does is self-perceived as not driven by power, allowing him to remain a mere bystander to the university's emetic activities.

At the end of the quote, Ramón deploys a local colloquialism to portray the power-seeking tactics at play within the university—the idea of accumulating or losing pins. *Chapas*, the actual word he uses, functions here as a metaphor for power by evoking the badges worn on someone's chest, such as those of a high-ranking military officer. The more pins one collects, the more power they signify—much like 'earning one's stripes' in Anglophone contexts. However, *chapa* is an overdetermined slang term. This is because it could also mean 'alias', like that of an undercover agent. Bearing this amphibology in mind, the way in which Ramón refers to himself and to his research—allegedly that university activity that does not truly belong to the university—is significant:

> I think the mafia-like university has always been that way, in the sense that loyalty is transient, so to speak. And I've been at the university for many years – I've got good friends at the university, so I work based on bonds of friendship. I'm not very instrumental in my work, you know? But since I've got little pins [*chapitas*] – and little pins [*chapitas*] are always valuable at the university – I can move; I can move around, you know? So, the co-researchers on my *fondecyt* project are more like friends I've been working with for a long time, and we have developed forms of loyalty, forms of… I don't know, even human protection. That is, regardless of whether someone is paid for a project, if it happens that one person ends up doing more work because someone else is dealing with other problems, that's fine.

All of a sudden, Ramón claims to be in possession of the very same asset that, in his view, has turned the university into a mafia. With a *slight* twist, however—he claims not to have proper pins, but petite ones: a miniaturised symbol of power. And what is that little pin of his? His *fondecyt*. This is the asset that makes him valuable to the university, as well as the enabler of his mobility. But, oddly enough, it is at the same time the feature that—if we are to remain consistent with his own speech—turns him into a discursive malefactor. After all, no matter how small the pins may be, they still count as pins. What seems to emerge here is the effort to sustain a fantasy of powerlessness. Ramón devotes considerable energy to distancing himself from the university's power games and, to achieve that, portrays himself as a kind of outsider from within, someone devoid of any desire for power. Despite his discursive contortions, his *fondecyt* is precisely where his speech trips over itself, revealing an attachment to power that was initially denied.

My interpretation here is that *fondecyts* introduce a short-circuit into Chilean academia, and that is precisely what the revolt brings to the fore. They bestow academics with a parcel of freedom—the mobility Ramón refers to—to conduct their research, a parcel over which they are the sole rightful owners. In the event of changing institutions, scholars 'take' their *fondecyts* with them. *Fondecyts*, then, represent a sort of juncture or hinge linking the university and its academics, albeit not entirely. This is why the act of researching, as we have seen, appears to occupy a unique and separate status from other 'positions' within the university. But this parcel of freedom is not without ambivalence. In the face of the galloping curtailment of academic freedoms brought about by the neoliberal reorganisation of the university, power has become almost anathema among academics, something persistently displaced. Let me offer just one concise example from a different participant. During a lesson in early June 2022, while speaking to her students about the *estallido*, Sofía remarked: 'The problem is not that academics speak, because power is not held by academics'. This encapsulates the fantasy that *fondecyt* enables *and* disrupts at once—namely, the narrative that power belongs exclusively to the Other. Ironically, these very products of the neoliberalisation of the university can act as an imaginary shield to which academics can resort in order to discursively detach themselves from the neoliberal university. It is a *small* parcel of power that, when set against the behemoth that is the university, *does not consciously register as power at all*.

In the most traditional psychoanalytic sense, *fondecyts* can be seen as a symptom of the Chilean neoliberal university—a substitutive formation of something that has been prevented from external manifestation. My view is that the predatory logics of the neoliberal university have had such a deep psychic impact on academics that some perceive themselves to be at the mercy of this unmitigatedly powerful institution. The fact that this is, in large part, a reasonable outcome of the university's current political economy does not, however, preclude a libidinal economy from running in parallel. In my interviews, what appears to follow *fondecyt* as its shadow is the fantasy of powerlessness—a defensive formation made, paradoxically, from the very composite that most academics try to distance themselves from: power. *Fondecyts* furnish academics with several expressions of power: money, legitimacy, prestige, stability, and, crucially, the possibility of constructing an 'extrinsic', non-neoliberalised parcel of their lives called 'my research'. Yet, since power within the university is unfailingly perceived as always-already neoliberal, it must be camouflaged. And perhaps this is why, of all things, Ramón resorts to the slang '*chapa*' to convey it: insofar as academic power cannot find external expression, it must circulate disguised—under an alias.

A Matter of Cookies

Let me provide another manifestation of this fantasy. A structural similarity with Ramón's account can be found in Cristina's. A significant portion of her speech revolved around the appointment to her current position. As she recounted, she felt that her presence was not particularly welcome from the outset. One of the main reasons for this, she believed, was that she arrived 'with the curriculum of the neoliberal generation of academics', that is, 'with *fondecyt* projects, publications, knowing English'. This situation, however, did not upset her, as she soon discerned that her disposition was markedly different from that of her colleagues. According to her, they all share a 'tiny, microscopic view' of what it means to have power within her faculty. In contradistinction, she holds a divergent understanding and vision of the university—one that, in her words, 'had left me out because I wasn't part of it; I wasn't friends with anyone here, and I wasn't interested in the same stuff'. At some point in the interview, she described the situation in the following terms:

> My stance was like: "Are you kidding me!?" I really couldn't believe people were fighting over this, cos it felt like just a little cookie [*galletita*] – the power of the faculty is a tiny cookie – and they showed such a lack of vision and understanding of the university as a whole.

Power in her faculty is a little cookie—sweet to some, but its flavour, it seems fair to infer, does not take Cristina's fancy. Surprisingly, this metaphor recurs throughout her speech. Almost every time she refers to her peers, she portrays them as ravenous cookie eaters, while she remains composed and detached. Her decision not to fight for the little cookie turned her into a pariah: 'They don't pay any attention to me. They don't include me when decisions are made – I'm nullified; I live on an island, you know? But for that very reason, I can do whatever I want'. The similarities between Ramón and Cristina are striking here: a) they both align with a negative perception of the university, one that reduces it to ruthless power games; b) they each proclaim to have no interest whatsoever in these power dynamics; and c) they seem to enjoy and take pride from their outcast status by seeking refuge in their research projects. Ultimately, since she has her research, Cristina is aware of the fact that 'the university doesn't end at the faculty, so I've got a whole world in which to grow, academically speaking'. For her, there seems to be a university beyond the university itself.

As a result of the *estallido*, Cristina claims, the quarrels over the tiny cookie did not cease, but they acquired a more human touch, so to speak. Her perception of her colleagues remained unchanged; however, she feels that the Department as a whole reached a deeper understanding of its members' biographies. Two months after the suspension of all academic activities at her university, a meeting was scheduled for the second half of November 2019. It would be the first time they had seen one another since the revolt began. The following is her recollection of what happened that day:

> I got up, and the meeting was, let's say, at nine. Lessons were suspended, of course, and I brought a cake [*un queque*], because I said: "It can't be like this; it can't be that we don't do something for each other", you know? I remember baking the cake [*hice el queque*], I put some chocolate

chunks in it, and I baked it just before leaving, so it arrived warm, with the chocolate pouring out (laughs).

Confectionery-based references, as we can see, permeate a good portion of Cristina's speech. Shortly after uttering that sentence, she set the two sweets in opposition: 'I must confess, I'm not into the tiny cookie; so if I had been, maybe I wouldn't have brought the cake'. We already know what the tiny cookie represents, so the question now is, what does the cake represent? In a way, it is what genuinely takes her fancy which, as she declares, academically speaking is her research. So, the first time they all reunited after the beginning of the revolt she decided—both metaphorically and literally—to put their differences on the table: she brought a bigger, more indulgent pudding to share with the tiny cookie eaters. Nonetheless, in yet another parallel with Ramón, her metaphor also backfires symbolically. In Chile, to bake a cake—*hacer un queque*—is a well-known idiom for adulation. The underlying logic is that someone's obsequious admiration for another is so strong that they are willing to go to great lengths in pursuit of that person's recognition. Of all things, then, that day she 'baked a cake' for her power-seeking colleagues—an act that can be read both as a symbolic gesture of distance *and* of concealed admiration.

What the fantasy of powerlessness reflects is the ambivalent status that power occupies within the neoliberal configuration of the Chilean university. It is no mystery that, in recent decades, the university has become, in many respects, an inhospitable place. Inhabiting the university and choosing to pursue an academic career are anything but straightforward decisions. Even for those comfortably situated within it, the inclination to decouple themselves from the logics of the contemporary university is entirely understandable. What perhaps comes as unexpected is the paradoxical manner in which some academics claim to achieve such a detachment. In my view, the overdetermined symbolic constructions of the little pins and the tiny cookie attest to the ambiguous and diminished status of academic power within the humanities and social sciences in Chile. Owing to a neoliberally propelled policy, *fondecyt* holders are able to construct a defensive narrative in which they are not totally part of the neoliberal university, since their only concern is their own research projects. Somehow, an activity unmistakably related to, and dependent on, the university is imaginarily reframed as a form of resistance against the university itself. In this context, power can only assume metonymic expressions.

The interpretation I propose here is that even in a context of rampant academic disempowerment—hitting particularly hard, it is worth noting, in the humanities and social sciences—powerlessness can nonetheless play an imaginary role. In a way, this is less counterintuitive than it might seem. In Chile, neoliberalism has eroded academic positions to such an extent that, for many, it appears that all that remains is to imaginarily redouble the wager: we have no more power to be dispossessed of; it is just me and my research—the Other holds all the power. However, as I have argued, *fondecyt* is a symptom—one of those things we cling to, no matter how much pain it provokes—insofar as it organises this fantasy despite being itself a symbol of power. From within this fantasy, it is as if, in resisting the largely oppressive power of the neoliberal university, *academics build a resistance to their own power*. And this might explain why, for those who embrace this fantasy, the *estallido* did not disrupt the logic of *fondecyt*: when research is imaginarily constructed as inherently non-neoliberal, or at least outside its circuits of power, academic writing becomes always-already an act of resistance. But, as I have tried to show here, resistance is not a piece of cake.

The Big Other's Desire

In 1977, Foucault (1980) engaged in a lengthy interview about Jeremy Bentham's idea of the panopticon and its revolutionary approach to surveillance. In his view, the critical innovation lies in its simplicity: where power once required costly physical and material constraints, after Bentham, all it takes is an inspecting gaze. The architecture of the panopticon permits an economisation of power—both in the sense of demanding fewer resources and in enabling the internalisation of this gaze, turning individuals into their own overseers. Through its conceptualisation as gaze, the scope of power expands almost infinitely, permeating the smallest particles of the social body. Simultaneously, power shifts from being identified with a sovereign who exercises it by right or birth to becoming 'a machine in which everyone is caught' (p. 156), a machine owned by no one. For Foucault, the panopticon describes a general system in utopian form, which leads him to draw an interest parallel with Rousseau:

> I would say Bentham was the complement to Rousseau. What in fact was the Rousseauist dream that motivated many of the revolutionaries? It was the dream of a transparent society, visible and legible in each of its parts, the dream of there no longer existing any zones of darkness, zones established by the privileges of royal power or the prerogatives of some corporations, zones of disorder. It was the dream that each individual, whatever position he occupied, might be able to see the whole of society [...]. Bentham is both that and the opposite. He poses the problem of visibility, but thinks of a visibility organised entirely around a dominating, overseeing gaze. He effects the project of a universal visibility which exists to serve a rigorous, meticulous power. Thus Bentham's obsession, the technical idea of the exercise of an "all-seeing" power, is grafted on to the great Rousseauist theme which is in some sense the lyrical note of the Revolution. (p. 152)

Let us fast-forward almost fifty years. According to Shoshana Zuboff (2023), we currently live in the age of surveillance capitalism. If industrial capitalism was characterised by its ability to transform nature's raw material into commodities, it is now human nature itself that is harnessed for a new market project. Far from the usual forms of capitalist exploitation, 'the essence of exploitation here is the rendering of our lives as behavioral data for the sake of others' improved control over us', where 'there is no exit, no voice, and no loyalty, only helplessness, resignation, and psychic numbing' (p. 204). We have been turned into means to the end of creating prediction products circulating in behavioural future markets. This accomplished version of the panopticon has no centre or identifiable agent, only an apparatus that Zuboff calls 'Big Other'. This apparatus is the offspring of neoliberalism and behaviourism, emerging through the reduction of human experience to measurable, observable units, with no concern for the meaning of that experience. For Zuboff, this way of knowing can be defined as 'radical indifference'—a form of 'observation without witness'. In this totalitarian picture, the anonymous Big Other operationalises this radical indifference:

> Big Other does not care what we think, feel, or do as long as its millions, billions, and trillions of sensate, actuating, computational eyes and ears can observe, render, datafy, and instrumentalize the vast reservoirs of behavioral surplus that are generated in the galactic uproar of connection and communication. (Zuboff, 2023, p. 206)

This indifference is tolerated insofar as the Big Other seizes our bodies for a seemingly non-violent regime, or at least significantly less visibly violent than in the past: we are exiled from our own behaviour, and we accept it. I am here less interested in the accuracy of this depiction of our contemporary world than in the underlying assumptions about how power operates. When we set aside the fact that the picture Zuboff paints is extraordinarily bleak, we can see that her approach aligns with the idea that power exists where things are made visible, and that the things which are visible are the only kinds of things that can exist in a given epoch (see Deleuze, 2018; and my discussion in Chapter 4). This means that, even if we do not agree with the image the Big Other produces of ourselves, this is the way in which we become visible in the present. The only option here, as Zuboff suggests, is to exercise autonomy; in other words, to resist predictability through *another type of visibility*. However, the irksome pebble in the shoe of this view is that we have no idea how individuals come to identify themselves with a regime of visibility, apart from the historical reconstruction that shows the power of the Big Other.

Following Todd McGowan (2018), the unresolved problem is that these accounts perform outstandingly well when it comes to theorising how power inserts itself into every aspect of the social, but cannot provide a satisfactory answer as to what drives people to accept it. For him, this is due to the exclusion of desire from these accounts—or, which amounts to the same, its inclusion merely as another cog in the power machine. Power, ironically, proves to be all too powerful, to the extent that it allows no internal contradiction, only external opposition. The result, as Joan Copjec (2015, p. 17) puts it, is that these (op)positional differences feed rather than threaten panoptic power, since the latter 'is ultimately *resistant to resistance*'. This is precisely the issue at stake in the fantasy of powerlessness. The pins and cookies show the libidinisation of power amid the revolt, which cannot be located either in compliance with the Big Other or in resistance through autonomy—they are an unconscious response to *the desire of the Other of the revolt*. This libidinisation has nothing to do with a 'capture' of desire by the managerial regime of academic performance; it is, rather, the proof that those positions are endemically incomplete, so subjects must imaginarily fill the gaps. Contrary Zuboff, the Other has always been indifferent to us, *and we cannot tolerate that*. That is why we keep trying to please it.

Ramón and Cristina do not fall into either the powerful or the powerless position; they use their power to construct an imaginary place of powerlessness where the misrecognition coming from the Other becomes endurable. They unconsciously deploy tangible expressions of power to present themselves *in the way they assume the Other wants to see them*: dispossessed of power. Their power must, therefore, find oblique ways of circulating in their speech, since a direct confrontation would undermine their imaginary security. Pins and cookies metonymically make power addressable; they allow it to be held while keeping it at arm's length. However, as per my interpretation, these signifiers exert their own autonomy, making explicit what they are meant to conceal: the camouflaging of power through an 'alias', in the case of Ramón; the adulation of the cookie eaters by 'baking them a cake', in the case of Cristina. When Rodrigo Nunes (2021) explores forms of immunity to political action, he notes that it is possible to exercise power without registering it as such. For him, this requires instituting two separate worlds: the first contains practices that are inherently compromised; the second is composed of practices that are corruptible exclusively from the outside. Ramón and Cristina produced precisely these two fantasmatic worlds to cope with the experience of the revolt. Within this fantasy, they can be powerfully powerless.

My interpretation corroborates Alenka Zupančič's (2016) assertion that the reason we are bound to discursive power lies primarily in its very flawed nature, not in its strength. In our subjection to power discourses—such as the managerial regime of performance in the university—there is always a 'redoubling' that is essential to their functioning.

Power must bridge its own internal gap in order to congregate individuals around it. For Zupančič, power is contingent not so much because it is open to the future—a future in which new positions of resistance might emerge—but because it is open to its own inconsistency. The unconscious redoubling of power, its sexualisation, is how this gap is filled. For psychoanalysis, sexuality is regarded as the propelling force of negativity:

> The truth is not that everything is sexual, but that there is something that can make anything sexual. Anything – including the act of copulation ("sexual intercourse") itself. And it is here, in this paradoxical redoubling, that we can perceive the structural gap which is conceptualized by psychoanalysis as that of the unconscious. (Zupančič, 2016, p. 61)

Do we not find a similar redoubling in the fantasy of powerlessness? The truth is not that everything is power, but that there is something that can render anything powerful—even the perception of an absence of power. This unconscious redoubling through sexualisation is what dominant approaches to power cannot accommodate. The Big Other of power, 'the puppet master' of surveillance capitalism (Zuboff, 2023, p. 206), has a missing string that makes it a *desiring* Other. The fantasy of powerlessness reveals this in the context of the *estallido*. Confronted with the call to live neoliberalism according to the logic of post-neoliberalism, the experiences of Ramón and Cristina illustrate the difficulty of navigating a politically empowering event when power is equated with neoliberalism. They responded to the emancipatory call of the revolt through an imaginary identification with powerlessness, a paradoxical unconscious solution to misrecognition that perpetuates the historical erosion of academics' power by means of managerial techniques. Within this fantasmatic formation, power is sexualised (redoubled) in order to construct a power-free zone where the empowering experience of the revolt can be sustained.

References

Araujo, K. (Ed.). (2019). *Hilos Tensados: Para Leer el Octubre Chileno*. Editorial Universidad de Santiago de Chile.

Balbontín, C., & Salas, R. (Eds.) (2020). *Evadir. La Filosofía Piensa la Revuelta de Octubre 2019*. Libros del Amanecer.

Ball, S. (Ed.). (2010). *Foucault and Education: Disciplines and Knowledge*. Routledge.

Ball, S. (2013). *Foucault, Power, and Education*. Routledge.

Besley, T., & Peters, M. (2007). *Subjectivity and Truth: Foucault, Education, and the Culture of Self*. Peter Lang.

Bevir, M. (Ed.). (2016). *Governmentality after Neoliberalism*. Routledge.

Brunner, J. (2015). Medio siglo de transformaciones de la educación superior chilena: Un estado del arte. In A. Bernasconi (Ed.), *La Educación Superior de Chile: Transformación, Desarrollo y Crisis*. Ediciones UC.

Callison, W., & Manfredi, Z. (Eds.). (2019). *Mutant Neoliberalism: Market Rule and Political Rupture*. Fordham University Press.

Cannizzo, F. (2018). Tactical evaluations: Everyday neoliberalism in academia. *Journal of Sociology, 54*(1), 77–91.

Clarke, J. (2017). So many strategies, so little time… making universities modern. In S. Hyatt, B. Shear & S. Wright (Eds.), *Learning Under Neoliberalism. Ethnographies of Governance in Higher Education*. Berghahn Books.

Copjec, J. (2015). *Read my Desire. Lacan Against the Historicists*. Verso.

Deleuze, G. (2018). *El Saber. Curso Sobre Foucault, Tomo 1*. Editorial Cactus.

Fardella, C., Sisto, V., & Jiménez, F. (2015). Nosotros los académicos. Narrativas identitarias y autodefinición en la universidad actual. *Universitas Psychologica, 14*(5), 1625–1636.

Foucault, M. (1980). The eye of power. In C. Gordon (Ed.), *Power/Knowledge: Selected Interviews and Other Writings by Michel Foucault, 1972–1977*. Pantheon Books.

Foucault, M. (2010). *The Birth of Biopolitics. Lectures at the Collège de France, 1978–1978*. Palgrave Macmillan.

Freud, S. (1991). *The Penguin Freud Library, Volume 1: Introductory Lectures on Psychoanalysis*. Penguin.

Henríquez, K., & Pleyers, G. (Eds.). (2023). *Chile en Movimientos*. CLACSO.

Kenny, J. (2018). Re-empowering academics in a corporate culture: An exploration of workload and performativity in a university. *Higher Education, 75*(2), 365–380.
Lemm, V., & Vatter, M. (Eds.). (2014). *The Government of Life: Foucault, Biopolitics, and Neoliberalism.* Fordham University Press.
Leyton, D. (2022). Neoliberalising working-class subjectification through affirmative action policies: Managerial leadership and ontological coaching in higher education. *Journal of Education Policy, 37*(3), 358–378.
Leyton, D., & Sánchez, G. (2024). Beyond (and alongside) shameful attachments: The lived experience of critique within the entrepreneurial university. *Cultural Studies ↔ Critical Methodologies, 24*(4), 251–262.
Majed, R. (2023). Sectarian neoliberalism and the 2019 uprisings in Lebanon and Iraq. In J. Karam & R. Majed (Eds.), *The Lebanon Uprising of 2019: Voices from the Revolution.* I.B. Tauris.
Marttila, T. (2018). Neoliberalism, the knowledge-based economy and the entrepreneur as metaphor. In D. Cahill, M. Konings, M. Cooper, & D. Primrose (Eds.), *The SAGE Handbook of Neoliberalism.* SAGE Publications.
McGowan, T. (2018). The sex in their violence: Eroticizing biopower. In V. Sinclair & M. Steinkoler (Eds.), *On Psychoanalysis and Violence: Contemporary Lacanian Perspectives.* Routledge.
Newfield, C. (2019). Innovation discourse and the neoliberal university: Top ten reasons to abolish disruptive innovation. In W. Callison & Z. Manfredi (Eds.), *Mutant Neoliberalism: Market Rule and Political Rupture.* Fordham University Press.
Nunes, R. (2021). *Neither Vertical nor Horizontal: A Theory of Political Organisation.* Verso.
Olssen, M. (2016). Neoliberal competition in higher education today: Research, accountability and impact. *British Journal of Sociology of Education, 37*(1), 129–148.
Olssen, M., & Peters, M. (2005). Neoliberalism, higher education and the knowledge economy: From the free market to knowledge capitalism. *Journal of Education Policy, 20*(3), 313–345.
Peters, M., & Jandrić, P. (2018). Neoliberalism and the university. In D. Cahill, M. Konings, M. Cooper, & D. Primrose (Eds.), *The SAGE Handbook of Neoliberalism.* SAGE Publications.
Rifo, M. (2017). Historia de la transformación en la educación superior chilena (1973-1990). *Revista Historia de la Educación Latinoamericana, 19*(28), 13–36.

Rose, N. (1996). *Inventing Our Selves: Psychology, Power, and Personhood*. Cambridge University Press.

Zuboff, S. (2023). The age of surveillance capitalism. In W. Longhofer & D. Winchester (Eds.), *Social Theory Re-Wired: New Connections to Classical and Contemporary Perspectives*. Routledge.

Zupančič, A. (2016). Biopolitics, sexuality and the unconscious. *Paragraph, 39*(1), 49–64.

8

Fantasies of Emancipation and Emancipatory Fantasies

My interrogation of the desire for social change in the Chilean revolt of 2019 was prompted by the dissatisfaction with the prevailing frameworks used to interpret it. As conceptualised in Chapter 1, the desire for social transformation is caught between restorative approaches, which understand emancipation as a means of regaining access to a non-estranged existence, and power-based models that aim to resist the oppressive technologies of historical modes of governmentality. Through these mutually reinforcing procedures, the desire for social change is persistently assumed to be an impulse that coincides with itself—a vitalist force that encounters only external opposition, preventing us from being who we truly are. I embarked on a study of the experience of the *estallido* to demonstrate the fragile foundations of this idea. As such, this book is less an analysis of the revolt itself than an exploration of the desire for social change within the context of the *estallido*. I am convinced that, if the Chilean revolt has any lessons to bequeath to future emancipatory movements, it is the confirmation that the desire for social change is an internally divided experience. The fantasies I have reconstructed in the previous chapters unequivocally demonstrate that, before confronting

G. Sánchez, *A Rebel Unconscious*, Studies in the Psychosocial,
https://doi.org/10.1007/978-3-032-12275-9_8

any external forces, those who embrace social change must first contend with the misrecognition produced by the emancipatory call of the revolt.

As Chapter 2 showed, there is ample conceptual evidence suggesting that the desire for social change is as ambivalent as any other desire. My aim was to provide empirical support for this claim. To that end, I conducted interviews and observations with critical academics committed to social transformation. Drawing on Simon Critchley's (2008) notion of ethical subjectivity, I defined them as *a way* of self-binding to a post-neoliberal society and the ongoing attempts to shape themselves in relation to this good. My definition avoided treating them as fully constituted subjects, allowing me to explore how they unconsciously negotiate, so to speak, their self-binding to the experience of the end of neoliberalism brought about by the revolt. Whether or not we can imagine individuals more committed to social change is beside the point. The objective was to show that even among intellectually and politically engaged individuals, there are symbolic negotiations that reveal the non-identical nature of the desire for emancipation. Most participants in my study had long anticipated an event of this kind, some even expressing surprise that it had not occurred sooner—the popular uprising was halfway between the desired and the foreseeable. And yet, as the preceding chapters have demonstrated, these committed individuals encountered considerable difficulties in recognising themselves within the new symbolic coordinates that emerged. The emancipatory interpellation of the Other of the *estallido* involved a dialectic of recognition and misrecognition that gave rise to a complex unconscious economy shaping the desire for change.

My goal in this final chapter is to draw the main conclusions of my study. First, I argue that my analysis corroborates the relevance of the notion of fantasy for the empirical study of emancipatory events and their identifications. In contrast to power-centred models, fantasy focuses on unconscious dynamics often overlooked in accounts of social change, particularly the ways in which we respond to our lack of self-identity. From there, I explore the commonalities across the five fantasies analysed, in order to distil some general patterns. Based on this exercise, I conclude that the emancipatory organisation of the revolt was lopsided: emancipatory meanings were largely underpinned by a neoliberal libidinal economy. Drawing on Todd McGowan's (2025) idea that what defines capitalism's psychic life is its rejection of limits through pure excess, I argue that there is substantial evidence to suggest that, to some extent, the psychic life of the revolt reproduced this same rejection. Finally, and in response to the premise of my research that there is no desire without a fantasmatic framework, I show how my interpretation of the revolt can contribute to the conceptualisation of emancipatory fantasies within contemporary psychoanalytic debates.

The Dignity of Fantasy

In May 2023, just as I was wrapping up my doctoral dissertation, a handful of colleagues and I had the opportunity to share a generous and intimate seminar with Jacqueline Rose at Birkbeck, University of London. Over the course of this exchange, she reflected on key moments in her intellectual journey, placing particular emphasis on political episodes that, in her own words, she simply could not walk away from. At some point, I asked her about a feature of her work that I have long admired: her ability to articulate politically progressive positions alongside the psychoanalytic notion of fantasy—a path that is, theoretically speaking, decidedly less travelled. Her reply was that she has always been interested in the question of what mobilises people to act, and especially in how they come to experience themselves as self-mobilised in the face of the inescapability of the unconscious. She then added: 'So, you have to fight for fantasy, because it has its dignity'. I wrote down this exact phrase in my notebook, and it has since prompted me to reflect on its resonance with the demand for dignity that emerged from the *estallido*. Fantasy has its dignity and the Chilean demand for dignity carries its own fantasies.

I bring up this recollection because turning to psychoanalysis to explore the subjective effects of an event like the Chilean revolt is an unconventional choice, even more so when it involves the notion of fantasy. As Roland Barthes (1985, p. 275) remarked to Bernard-Henri Lévy in an interview, the imaginary is 'almost the poor relation of psychoanalysis […], it seems underrated, at least by the psychoanalytic vulgate'.

If one wishes to demonstrate their critical credentials from a psychoanalytic point of view, there are more fashionable candidates for the task. The register of the real and its satellite concepts—drive and *jouissance*, for instance—have long been the default options when invoking Lacan to interpret social phenomena. According to Lacan, the real is the impossible: 'Not in the name of a simple obstacle we hit our heads up against, but in the name of the logical obstacle of what, in the symbolic, declares itself to be impossible. This is where the real emerges from' (Lacan, 2007, p. 123). The parallels between the dislocatory effects of the *estallido* and the kind of impossibility described by the real are evident: the revolt was not a simple obstacle we stumbled into, but an actual impossibility for the continued reproduction of our lives as we had lived them until then.

The main problem with this approach is that it applies psychoanalytic theory to explain the *estallido*, rather than to explore it (e.g., Uribe, 2020). In doing so, it ends up domesticating an event that is, ironically, framed as impossible. It is almost as if reading Lacan were all one needed to understand the revolt; as though Lacanian psychoanalysis were inherently anti-neoliberal (e.g., Dureuil, 2023). Moreover, even if the logic behind this approach were not reductionist, its outcome can only lead to a stalemate. The question we should pose is simple: what is gained by claiming that the *estallido* is the 'real', unsymbolisable element of Chile's democratic history? Beyond a kind of intellectual self-reassurance, not much. As soon as a sociopolitical event is conflated with a concept, interpretations are foreclosed. Ultimately, as Anna Kornbluh (2022, p. 35) sharply observes: 'Overly romantic notions of the real in psychoanalytic political theory omit the dialectical character of the real's constitution by the symbolic'.

Furthermore, the decision to extract a snippet of Lacan's theory in order to explain events such as the revolt runs counter to Lacan's own position; he consistently maintained that psychoanalysis does not offer the key to the universe. Rather, psychoanalysis 'is governed by a particular aim, which is historically defined by the elaboration of the notion of the subject. It poses this notion in a new way, by leading the subject back to his signifying dependence' (Lacan, 1998, p. 77). This was the starting point of my research. I argued that there is sufficient evidence to support the claim that the *estallido* represented a post-neoliberal mode of organising social life in Chile, and that such an emancipatory organisation was symbolic in nature. Drawing on Jacques Rancière (2010), I suggested that the revolt enabled Chileans to experience neoliberalism through the logic of post-neoliberalism. Accordingly, I conceptualised the *estallido* as the Other that made this emancipatory experience accessible, in order to explore the unconscious economy of the desire for social change. My analysis focused strategically on critical academics, as they can be treated as subjects who attempt to shape themselves in accordance with the good of social change (Critchley, 2008). Consequently, my research is a psychoanalytically inspired study of the Chilean revolt not because it offers a Lacanian explanation of the event, but because it takes seriously the symbolic nature of the *estallido*. This has allowed me to explore its unconscious mediations and, in doing so, to grasp a dimension of the desire for social change that is obfuscated by power-centred models: its internally divided nature as an experience.

Based on the above, the perspective I adopted in this book sought to do justice to the 'dignity of revolt' advanced by Julia Kristeva (2025). For her, the revolt is a moment marked by a 'retrospective return' in which the subject is able to question its own truth. Kristeva puts forward a notion of revolt grounded in the Freudian discovery of the unconscious, which implies that such an event cannot be understood without acknowledging the permanence of contradiction. In her view, even in an era where true revolts are increasingly rare, 'we can still contemplate the rebellious potentialities that the imaginary might resuscitate in our innermost depths' (Kristeva, 2025, p. 14). Revolt and the imaginary go hand in hand. This resonates with Kornbluh's (2019, p. 164) assertion that 'any analysis of social transformation must address psychic transformation'. I operationalised this psychic transformation in terms of fantasy. The 'real', dislocatory nature of the *estallido* is thus taken as the background against which a new field of discursivity emerges, a process that gives rise to new symbolic practices and, as a corollary, new imaginary stabilisations of meaning and recognition. If, as Manuel Canales (2022) suggests in the title of his book, Chile's revolt arises in the form of a question, it is because the *estallido* reorganised the social bond in Chile through an interpellative call to live neoliberalism according to the logic of post-neoliberalism.

The above is both a factual corroboration and a theoretical principle. On the one hand, the protests that preceded the revolt on 18 October—high school students jumping over turnstiles at tube stations—and the actions that followed did not take place in the desert of the real. On the contrary, they offered a range of discursive elements—mottoes, rationales, and narratives—that people could draw on to forge a counter-hegemonic identity. The fact that I was able to reconstruct five fantasies organising unconscious responses to the revolt's question corroborates the symbolic nature of the experience of the end of neoliberalism and the impossibility of arriving at a single, 'correct' answer. On the other hand, this also points to the inescapability of the imaginary realm in our lives. As Calum Neill (2013, p. 339) succinctly puts it, 'there is no experience of the world which is not affected by identification'. To acknowledge that the revolt was even minimally meaningful is already to accept, tacitly, its imaginary dimension; namely, the fact that subjects sustain this new experience of the world through fantasmatic investments.

For reasons I can only speculate about, within the community of scholars who draw on the notion of fantasy for empirical research, there is a marked selectivity in how the concept is deployed. As discussed in the first chapters of this book, despite widespread acknowledgement of the inexorability of the imaginary realm in the structuration of meaning (Ffytche, 2019; Glynos, 2011; Neill, 2013), academic attention tends to 'naturally' gravitate towards politically undesirable forms of identification. Put differently, fantasy is most often treated as a cog in the machinery of power and domination, a crucial mechanism for the camouflaging of oppression. The consequences of this are twofold. First, it produces a theoretical impasse: an ontological premise (all identifications rely on a fantasmatic scaffolding) is filtered through an epistemological narrowing (oppressive identifications receive disproportionate scrutiny). Second, it fosters a false sense of clarity when it comes to politically progressive identifications. To the extent that fantasy is presumed to operate solely within power dynamics, emancipatory or counter-hegemonic identifications are implicitly construed as unfolding in a fantasy-free zone. Otherwise, and this is the point I wish to emphasise, we would be forced to accept that the desire for social change and its identifications are just as contradictory and messy as all the others.

My study has shown that fantasies are unavoidable when approaching emancipatory experiences. Their dignity in the field of social change lies in their capacity to capture the diverse ways in which subjects can respond to the misrecognition of the Other. In this sense, repression by no means exhausts our psychic life. As the interpretation developed in previous chapters evinces, confronting structural alienation can bring our most creative capacities to the fore. Elements of our experience of the end of neoliberalism may indeed be repressed, but they may also be openly acknowledged and simultaneously denied, exist without counting, count without existing, be performed while remaining impossible, or be embraced while kept at a distance. All of this is possible because these experiences are underpinned by a libidinal economy. Such an economy takes the form of unconscious circuits of excess and antagonism that accompany our conscious practices (Kapoor et al., 2023; Kapoor, 2020) and can be reconstructed by tracing the autonomy of the signifier. The recognition of recognition, that crucial step in the process of identification outlined in Chapter 2, can take all these contradictory forms—and many others my study did not manage to capture—because the non-neoliberal words that held so much meaning during the revolt (Castillo, 2019) were sustained by imaginary investments. Without fantasies, we simply cannot account for this dimension of our desire for social change.

I approached the revolt on the assumption that the array of new symbolic associations it set in motion required a fantasmatic cushioning on the part of the subject. All I did, then, was to apply to the investigation of the desire for emancipation the same interpretive principles that have guided some of the most rigorous studies on the logic of fantasy in other fields (e.g., McMillan, 2017; Ronderos & Glynos, 2022; Sánchez et al., 2024; Seitz & Proudfoot, 2021; Vadolas, 2012). In order to show that the identification with counter-hegemonic discourses is anything but an immediate or straightforward process—as the relative lack of scholarly attention to this question might suggest—I explored its vicissitudes among critical academics. This group emerges as one of the collectives most likely to expect a direct correlation between subject positions and the desire for social transformation. For people whose desire appears to be almost naturally directed towards the good of social change, radical transformation should, in theory, have felt like an experience of self-recognition. At the unconscious level, however, my study shows that the waters are far muddier than this reasonable yet idealised portrayal would suggest.

Excessive Responses to Excess

The five fantasies I reconstructed in the preceding chapters point precisely to the psychic difficulties involved in identification with the *estallido*. In this section, I would like to group them according to their commonalities in order to derive some structural challenges. The fantasies of sleeplessness and immediacy primarily concern the visual field of the revolt, representing two poles of the same experience. At their most basic, the fantasies of impotence, clairvoyance, and powerlessness take the act of writing as their referent. Grouping the fantasies according to these experiential domains makes it easier to perceive their shared psychic structure. For example, the fantasies related to the visuality of the revolt clearly expose the magnitude of the subjective costs people had to bear in order to keep pace with its unfolding. To a large extent, this was an unintended outcome of the *estallido*'s contingency—an undirected event propelled by an anonymous yet pressing force. These fantasies appear to execute opposite manoeuvres and consequently aim to achieve different goals. Interestingly, however, they turn out to be merely separate ways of doing exactly the same thing: coping with what they perceive the revolt demands from the subject. In both cases, the *estallido* is internalised as an injunction not to be duped. This point deserves further comment.

One of the most distinctive tenets of the discourse surrounding the revolt is the idea that its emergence marks a turning point in the country's self-consciousness: we used to believe we were doing fine, but now *we can see* how things really are. And we can see because *we are no longer asleep*. At a symbolic level, the misperception of the lived situation is not due to a political obstacle as such but rather to the vital function of resting. Accordingly, we can now perceive the reality of our oppression and act upon it because we sleep no more. It follows from this that the Chilean people were 'a sleeping but sovereign *demos* that woke up' to retrieve 'the founding experience of equality that feeds the secret life of every democracy' (López, 2021, p. 22). In such a context, the symbolic manifestations on the street can be understood as 'a reminder of the many reasons why Chile should never "fall asleep" again' (De Vivanco & Johansson, 2021, p. 12). For many, these could be dismissed as nothing more than rhetorical vehicles for mobilising a deeper truth; symbolic ornaments crafted to embellish the revolt's actual message. Both my approach and interpretation suggest otherwise.

By linking the act of awakening with the possibility of overcoming the current state of domination, falling asleep was inadvertently rendered equivalent to the perpetuation of the neoliberal yoke—and thus, we should refrain from anything that might make us drowsy. In this scenario, tiredness becomes semantically and experientially indistinguishable from being wrong. That the command to never fall asleep again is not a mere decorative supplement is evident in the problematic place that truth occupies in the two fantasies about seeing. The fantasies of sleeplessness and immediacy stage psychic solutions to the quandary elicited by an interpellative call that hinges on vigilance and concentration. In this context, the subject must devise fantasmatic responses to the excessive demand of the revolt, which calls for an indefatigable and disproportionate attentiveness in return. Whether through an identification with the Other to avoid succumbing to somnolence, or through the Herculean task of recording every act at all times, individuals cling to certain signifiers to remain on the right side, that is, permanently awake. When truth is visible and nothing obstructs our view of it, vision is elevated to a moral duty.

The psychic *cul-de-sac* of the revolt in the field of vision shares an intriguing parallel with what William Mazzarella (2017) identifies as the fantasy of perfect addressability. In his analysis of contemporary marketing and media, Mazzarella refers to the impact of neurosciences and digital algorithms on the construction of the subject they seek to produce. What these technologies appear to herald is the waning of the assumption that, beneath the layers of manipulation characteristic of mass publicity, we might still find an autonomous subject irreducible to such strategies. The point is that nowadays, thanks to a level of customisation and narrowcasting unthinkable even a decade ago, we seem to be addressed as exactly who we are. Perfect addressability, then, names 'a situation in which there is no perceptible gap between the media that address me and my innermost understandings of myself' (Mazzarella, 2017, p. 109). I would like to suggest that an equivalent dynamic can be found in the *estallido*. To put it directly: once full visibility becomes mandatory and not seeing is taken as a sign of weakness or oppression, then the only possible interpellation—or addressability, in Mazzarella's terms—is *perfect* interpellation. At a scopic level, the revolt allows no room for interruption or intermittence, so fantasies become imaginary solutions to this demand.

Based on the above, the fantasies around seeing (during) the *estallido* are transindividual scenarios that help subjects imaginarily sustain the excessiveness of the revolt *through more excess*. When we pay attention to the symbolic structuration of the revolt's visual field, we can appreciate how its unconscious economy appears to operate a reversal of the neoliberal one—a reversal yet not a transformation. The soporific effects of neoliberalism, according to the narrative, were permanent: Chileans were uninterruptedly asleep, incapable of seeing their subjugation. The analeptic properties of the *estallido* produce the same result, only in the opposite way: we are now always awake, permanently able to see the actual state of affairs. Discursively, the popular uprising gave rise to meanings and practices opposed to the neoliberal configuration of everyday life. At an unconscious level, however, the revolt seemed to fall back on the libidinal economy already in place. What I suggest is that the *estallido* did not lessen the psychic strains of neoliberalism in order to mobilise these new meanings; rather, it attempted to make use of the excess in a non-neoliberal fashion. Therefore, at least in the terrain of visibility, the revolt did not significantly alter the unconscious circuit of neoliberalism but instead channelled it in a different direction. Rather than relaxing the tightness of the previous grip, the Chilean awakening forced the subject to double down on this logic.

Let me now turn to the fantasies pertaining to the act of writing. These stage the psychic labour required to navigate power and capacity amid the experience of the end of neoliberalism. Some individuals experienced a sudden inability to perform the quintessential task of writing; others felt that their previous status had been unjustly eroded, rendering their writing meaningless; and still others perceived themselves as stripped of all institutional power, seeking shelter in writing instead. All of this is veridical, first and foremost, at an imaginary level—they lose power within the fantasies that allow them to experience reality, but not necessarily outside this libidinal framework. Based on their own accounts, these subjects *do* write, *do* retain their scholarly status, and *do* exert power within the university, and yet they appear to access their desire only by perceiving themselves as dispossessed from most forms of power. Whether in an oblique or explicit fashion, the neoliberal Other is invariably portrayed as the greedy entity hoarding all the power. The privileged place that loss occupies in these fantasies may help explain why 'othering' certain fictitious or real groups emerges as the main source of unconscious satisfaction. These others are seen as extracting some kind of corrupt enjoyment from their transgressive behaviour, something inaccessible to those engaged in the fantasising. The crucial point is that, of course, the accusers partake in the very same activities they claim to reject, which leads them to rehearse sometimes extreme imaginary contortions in order to accommodate this situation.

Lacan (2020) refers to the unconscious as the inverted message the subject receives from the Other. This is an unknown message as it becomes captured by the imaginary relationship between the ego and the other (human being)—a relation set in motion precisely to obstruct the recognition of this inverted and unwanted message, which contains the unconscious truth of the subject's desire. By fixating desiring scenarios, fantasy functions as a defence against this unconscious truth. As I have mentioned, these scenarios construct an other that is crucial to their maintenance, but they also create modes of access to objects. In their speech, the participants of my study talk about many such objects and their particular ways of accessing them: books, articles, *fondecyts*, universities, research centres, and so on. The singularity of Lacanian psychoanalysis lies in the idea that what propels the subject's relationship with the world is the primordial lack of the object, a lack that carries not a negative but a productive connotation. Lacan identifies three 'terms of reference' for the lack of the object, which might illuminate certain aspects of the fantasies outlined in my interpretation.

Symbolic indebtedness is the first term. In relation to castration, Lacan suggests that what is lacking is not a real, factual object. The object of symbolic castration is always imaginary—the phallus, that mythical guarantor of full meaning. In its absence, symbolic indebtedness is the way in which the subject recognises the law and punishment. In the second term, imaginary detriment, the object is 'well and truly real' but the frustration or lack is 'wholly imaginary'. The singularity of frustration lies in the fact that the subject aspires to be vindicated and feels entitled to demand the object. When frustrated, the subject feels deprived of the object by someone else but—and here is the imaginary twist—this is experienced as a withdrawal of love: what is lacking is the love bestowed by the other through the gift. In the final term of reference, privation, we encounter the lack of a symbolic object. This is premised on the corroboration that, in the world, nothing lacks in itself unless symbolised. We can only form the idea that something is not in its place once both that something and that place have been coated in signifiers; otherwise, it would not hold. The paradigmatic form of privation is the woman's lack of a penis. In reality, of course, the woman does not lack anything; we only get the idea that she does if, through the introduction of some kind of symbolic law, we establish that something should be in a certain place (Chiesa, 2007).

I argue that we can draw compelling correlations between these three terms of reference for the lack of the object and the three fantasies related to power. For the sake of clarity, I shall proceed schematically.

- Symbolic indebtedness appears as a way of understanding what is at stake in the fantasy of impotence. In this scenario, as we saw, Carlos and Cristina are not impotent in the way they claim; that is, they do not lack a factual object (a missing potency). Furthermore, particularly in Carlos' experience, what they seem to desire is the Law—a Law capable, for instance, of effectively separating genuine scholars from other, bogus academics. Ultimately, Carlos and Cristina sacrifice their knowledge to put the Other to work, restoring an imaginary pre-castration moment.

- The fantasy of clairvoyance strongly echoes the logic of frustration. It can be said that the lack experienced in both Carmen's and Sofía's accounts relates to a real, veridical object: they genuinely did not know about the *estallido* in advance, and neither of them was able to warn others about what was to come. So, irrespective of the impossibility of this task, the object is factual, yet the lack is clearly imaginary. In a peculiar dialectic, the triumph of sociology is unconsciously registered as a loss: the dissemination of sociological tools feels subjectively harmful. Introducing the logic of frustration allows us to consider that this may be the case because what Carmen and Sofía experience is a withdrawal of love: the revolt took place and, as a result, they were no longer the sole recipients of public attention as they once were.
- Finally, a parallel can be drawn between the privation of the object and the fantasy of powerlessness. What Ramón and Cristina share is a conscious refusal of power *tout court*, which they consistently locate within the neoliberal university. Through the liminal nature of their research grants, they are able to construct a fantasy of a non-neoliberalised space they can inhabit without partaking in the university—despite, in fact, being fully part of it. In a manner of speaking, their speeches resemble the belief that the woman actually lacks a penis: they perceive themselves—and construct their fantasmatic scenarios accordingly—on the assumption that academics *should renounce power altogether*. Interestingly, what is perpetuated in this fantasy, through the appearance of resistance, is the very symbolic delimitation of power established by the neoliberal Other, the underlying reason for their disempowerment.

Over thirty years ago, Ernesto Laclau (1990) identified the problems that the notion of power poses to the theorisation of emancipatory movements. The widely accepted premise that identities are forged antagonistically—namely, that sustaining what something is inevitably involves defining what it is not—may lead progressive positions to assume that the emancipatory goal is the suppression of power. Given its relevance to my argument, I will quote almost the entire passage:

> Underlying that response is the assumption that a free society is one from which power has been totally eliminated. But as we saw, if power is the prerequisite of any identity, the radical disappearance of power would amount to the disintegration of the whole social fabric. [...] it is this profound contradiction which underlies any project of *global* emancipation. By global emancipation we do not mean specific or even a broad and articulated set of emancipations, but the notion of an emancipation aimed at transforming the very "root" of the social. A harmonious society is impossible because power is the condition for society to be possible (and at the same time, impossible [...]). Even in the most radical and democratic projects, social transformation thus means building a new power, not radically eliminating it. Destroying the hierarchies on which sexual or racial discrimination is based will, at some point, always require the construction of other exclusions for collective identities to be able to emerge. (Laclau, 1990, p. 33)

What Laclau identifies as the profound contradiction of emancipatory projects has more recently been discussed by Vladimir Safatle (2022) in terms of the belief that all external causality is always-already oppression. While the dilemma of heteronomy does indeed have important implications for the conceptualisation of emancipatory projects, my study shows that this profound contradiction is not merely conceptual but experiential. My interpretation demonstrates that the way in which this contradiction is imaginarily 'solved' is of upmost importance. The belief that power and neoliberalism are synonymous results in an unconscious rejection of negativity that severely curtails the emancipatory potential of the *estallido*. In one way or another, when confronted with the desiring call to live neoliberalism according to the logic of post-neoliberalism, individuals turned partial lack into excess: they were *fully* incapable of doing something they did, *fully* deprived of the love of the public, *fully* dispossessed of power. As in the fantasies of the scopic field, here the excess of the call was met with more excess.

'The promise of capitalism', McGowan (2025, p. 27) maintains, 'is that the excess of the commodity can cure us of our lack'. The fantasies I have reconstructed in this book follow a similar pattern: the excess of the *estallido* can cure us of our lack. The unconscious investment in this idea is what, at times, brought the revolt dangerously close to the neoliberal fantasy. For McGowan, the psychic allure of capitalism derives from its rejection of limits by staging a fantasy of pure excess. This is the source of the commodity's appeal despite its permanent failure: it creates the illusion that we can eliminate the boundaries of our experience and perceive ourselves as whole. My suggestion that certain elements of the revolt represent a significant continuity of the neoliberal libidinal economy follows from this idea. There is a fantasmatic dimension of the *estallido* that was mobilised to sustain an experience of self-identity that, even when expressed in emancipatory terms, mirrored the neoliberal fantasy of pure excess. The conscious rebellion against the neoliberal organisation of life successfully rejected its meanings but, at least to some extent, preserved its unconscious rejection of limits. In this study, the different scenarios framing the desire for social change are tied together by a single impulse: to combat misrecognition through fantasies of a non-lacking excess. It is precisely this impulse that a rebel unconscious disrupts.

The *estallido* was the most empowering sociopolitical event that Chile experienced in its recent democratic history, and perhaps in its entire existence as an independent country. Never before has a spontaneous expression of popular power reached such heights. This transformation, nevertheless, was accompanied by significant libidinal continuity. My interrogation of the desire for social change is consistent with Freud's (1981, p. 244) claim that 'it is a matter of general observation that people never willingly abandon a libidinal position, not even, indeed, when a substitute is already beckoning to them'. The transformative symbolic life of the *estallido*, as I have shown, was materially underway from the outset. But attaining recognition within this new symbolic environment required confronting structural misrecognition. Neoliberalism was not merely an obstacle to a better life but a *cherished* obstacle—something that could not be dispensed with without simultaneously abandoning a libidinal position. This position is driven by the fantasy of pure excess, and my exploration has demonstrated the various ways in which it paradoxically supported the experience of the end of neoliberalism. In the end, my interrogation of the desire for social change further illuminates the 'necessarily unsynchronised relationship between psychic and social transformation' that Hannah Proctor (2024, p. 19) identified in similar emancipatory experiences.

Emancipatory Fantasies?

It follows from the previous section that the fantasies framing the desire for social change presented in this book stress a paradox: the *estallido* produced meanings that challenged—and even temporarily replaced—certain neoliberal understandings while retaining some of their libidinal mainstays. At times, it even took advantage of them. My study, of course, does not exhaust the unconscious richness of the *estallido*, but it nonetheless shows how some of its crucial transformative components remained in solidarity with neoliberalism. And this is precisely where the notion of fantasy proves its dignity. By focusing on the lateral symbolic associations that emerge in subjects' attempts to convey meaning, we can identify the imaginary economies undergirding this process. This is what allows us to perceive the resilience of the neoliberal libidinal economy against the backdrop of 'phrases that neoliberalism cannot understand, but which are full of meaning for the revolt' (Castillo, 2019, p. 41). In other words, the existence and circulation of transformative meanings do not necessarily imply a change in the unconscious life of the regime being challenged—opposite meanings can, in some cases, be buttressed by identical unconscious dynamics.

The foregoing conclusion offers us a clue to understanding the vertiginous unfolding of events in Chile since October 2019. A quick glance at the country today is enough to make one believe the *estallido* never occurred. In a shockingly short period, not only was the spirit of the revolt crushed, but it would not be an exaggeration to claim that every political triumph was reversed. One fine morning, the Chilean people were burning the country down; suddenly, everything seemed possible. We subsequently found ourselves on the brink of having the most progressive constitution in the world, to be issued under the leadership of the youngest and most radical president since 1990. Four years later, the constitutional draft was rejected, a second failed process was led by a far-right coalition, the young radical president became a timid reformist, and everything that now seems possible is once again shaped by the neoliberal aegis. How can a country that has been rocked by such a radical sociopolitical event so easily return to business as usual after only a few years?

Based on my interpretation, trying to find an answer at the level of meaning would be to no avail. It is not so much that the revolt's discourse was too ambitious or not radical enough to defy the prevailing one. The point, rather, is that the transformation of neoliberal meanings was not accompanied by an equivalent transformation of its libidinal economy. The role played by negativity, as emphasised in this book, is the most palpable example of this—and, simultaneously, the most overlooked dimension of the revolt. The tenacity of power-centred models and the restorative approach severely obstructs the acknowledgement of this fact. From this point of view, the *estallido* 'marked an uprising of the nation's leftovers as they claimed their presence in a Chilean sociopolitical landscape that was designed to deny them any institutionally validated agency' (Woods, 2022, p. 167). A change in the sociopolitical landscape will allow 'the nation's leftovers' to regain cultural recognition; that, supposedly, is what the revolt was all about. If this were not accomplished, it was either due to the limitations of discourse in addressing all the 'leftovers' or to the resistance of established powers. The silence surrounding the structural misrecognition embedded in the search for a non-neoliberal identification is, however, deafening. This silence impedes us from seeing how the *estallido* was as psychically excessive as neoliberalism, thereby reducing the psychic cost of reverting to a previous meaning formation once the experience of the end of neoliberalism began to wane.

The interpretation offered in this book confirms the theoretical premise that there is no unconscious desire without a fantasmatic narrative organising it, regardless of how progressive that desire might be. Consequently, there should be a way of discriminating between conservative and progressive fantasies. Some Lacanian authors, however, stand against this idea. Lee Edelman (2007) is one of the most prominent. He advocates for something akin to a post-fantasmatic politics—effectively, a post-political scenario—which, for him, is a desirable outcome. Edelman maintains that the historicity of desire finds its temporalisation in politics; that is, its translation into a teleological narrative. From his perspective, fantasy cannot be emancipatory, insofar as politics confers social viability upon the succession of our libidinal attachments, thus occluding the negativity of the social:

> Politics, that is, by externalizing and configuring in the fictive form of a narrative, allegorizes or elaborates sequentially, precisely as desire, those overdeterminations of libidinal positions and inconsistencies of psychic defenses occasioned by what disarticulates the narrativity of desire: the drives, themselves intractable, unassimilable to the logic of interpretation or the demands of meaning-production; the drives that carry the destabilizing fore of what insists outside or beyond, because foreclosed by, signification. (Edelman, 2007, p. 9)

For Edelman, a queer project should resist the temptation of becoming something, that is, it must reject imaginary identifications and directly 'embody' its impossibility (the real). As Mari Ruti (2018) shows, the sheer antisociality of this position equates destructiveness with the ethical. In this book, I have argued that such a paradigm cannot serve as the sole yardstick for judging the desire for social change. Edelman's interpretation of politics as the temporalisation of the historicity of desire is indeed correct, yet his conclusions are debatable. His position is ultimately untenable in theoretical terms, since his account gives the impression that we can choose between the registers of the symbolic, the imaginary, and the real. Lacanian psychoanalysis maintains that human experience can only transpire within these registers, not that one is preferrable to the other. We do not experience the real, then a bit of symbolisation, and subsequently a pinch of the imaginary. This misreading of psychoanalytic theory leads to one-size-fits-all accounts of social change that are of little help in understanding emancipatory events like the *estallido*.

My psychoanalytic approach to the desire for social change runs counter to the idea that the ultimate goal of emancipation is desubjectivation. What we find in some versions of power-centred models, and even in certain Lacanian approaches, are the alleged 'politico-ethical benefits of subjective pulverization and radical antinormativity' (Ruti, 2018, p. 53). Despite their theoretical influences, these hyperbolic accounts of the desire for social change seem, perhaps surprisingly, to rely on a solid notion of the subject: the latter comes first, and political movements are expected to dissolve it. In contrast, Lacanian psychoanalysis posits a productive negativity. As Alenka Zupančič maintains:

> [...] when one speaks about desubjectivation or subjective destitution, we must not make the mistake of thinking that you start with a subject and then you have a whole movement to destitute it and then you're left with what? This is a mistake. Destitution of the subject *precedes* subjectivity. You don't start with subject and then go about its dismantling. It is not as if whatever subjectivity there is, it is there on behalf of the destitution. The notion of the subject is related to this radical negativity, but it isn't as if we have to destitute the subject, as if we are persons and then we have to destitute ourselves. (Zupančič & Terada, 2015, p. 196)

The fact that the destitution of the subject precedes subjectivity means that, regardless of how successful an emancipatory movement may be, *there is something we cannot get rid of*. This, nonetheless, should not lead us to believe that immobility is the only option once we accept that our subjectivity cannot be entirely dismantled. What Zupančič points to is that subjective liquidation can only produce fantasmatic getaways, since such efforts attempt to eradicate the very condition of emancipatory commitments: the negativity of the subject. As she insists: 'It is not as if first we get rid of something. On the contrary, it is through this radical negativity that something appears' (Zupančič & Terada, 2015, p. 196). If we do not want to fall prey to the allures of irrepresentability and destruction, as Kornbluh (2022) observes, we must acknowledge the importance of the signifying function for political activity. This, in turn, implies that there must be a way to conceptualise emancipatory fantasies.

Ruti (2012, 2017, 2018) offers a way to do this. From her perspective, Lacanian psychoanalysis allows us to understand defiant subjects in terms of the kind of desire they choose to pursue. Accepting that the mediation of the Other is unavoidable for the subject to exist, she argues that this is not an impediment but the very condition of social change. The fact that we learn to desire through the fantasmatic narratives addressing the desire of the Other means, in turn, that the Other does not know what its desire is either. This opens up the possibility of a desire that is not directly at the service of the existing order. Lacan's (1998, p. 214) claim that 'the desire of the Other is apprehended by the subject in that which does not work' points precisely in that direction.

This approach does not deny that fantasies entail alienation. However, the crucial point is that they simultaneously enable a subjective *separation* from the desire of the Other. This is the rather counterintuitive political potential of fantasies for Ruti: from within alienation in socially constructed fantasies, we can access our fundamental fantasies, those 'deposits of desire that are more representative of our singularity than what we inherit from the Other' (Ruti, 2012, p. 79). From this angle, a subject of ethical capacity does not emerge from the shattering of symbolic representation—as Edelman maintains—but from its lack of foundations. Consequently, 'the point is to peel off some of the layers of social conditioning so as to allow us to access forms of desire that might evade the demands of both conventional morality and economic exigency' (Ruti, 2018, p. 108). Fantasies, thus, challenge the widespread assumption that emancipation is a matter of overcoming alienation. The latter is unavoidable if we aspire to retain a minimal level of sociality, and yet we can still rebel against oppressive social arrangements—not by negating the desire of the Other but by separating ourselves from it.

This way of understanding the political potential of fantasies represents an alternative to the antisocial or purely disruptive accounts of the desire for social change within Lacanian scholarship. However, it still rests on two tricky premises. First, that 'the fundamental fantasy resides beyond the reach of the signifier' (Ruti, 2010, p. 10), which introduces a hierarchy of fantasies and situates some of them in a relatively mystical realm. Second, and particularly important for my enterprise, that the emancipatory potential of fantasies lies in their capacity to separate us from the desire of the Other. Implicit here is the assumption that the Other is always and invariably oppressive. In the context of this book, we should ask ourselves: is separation still the emancipatory way forward when the Other stands for the progressive organisation of the social bond? Or can fantasy *itself* be emancipatory? This is the challenge the *estallido* poses to a Lacanian approach to the desire for social change.

Todd McGowan maintains that fantasies can indeed be emancipatory. His approach explicitly challenges the idea that 'emancipation appears to hit a roadblock in fantasy' and that, consequently, the goal of political movements is 'to eviscerate this barrier' (McGowan, 2022, p. 177). In this vein, he distinguishes between emancipatory and conservative fantasies. The latter seeks to isolate enjoyment by positing a discontinuity between fantasy and social reality: the agent who enjoys does not belong to society and becomes an external threat to it. In contradistinction, emancipatory fantasies reject this disjunctive relationship with the social reality. 'The emancipatory project', McGowan (2022, p. 180) claims, 'constrains the subject to recognize its own involvement in the enjoyment that it fantasizes about'. What separates conservative from emancipatory fantasies is the fact that the former do not allow fantasy to intrude into social reality, thereby sustaining an ideological distance. This turns fantasy into a manoeuvre to spatialise the antagonistic character of the social and externalise it. Conversely, a fantasy can be regarded as emancipatory insofar as it intrudes into the social, enabling the subject to see itself within the fantasy.

Thus conceived, fantasies are not problematic because they channel libidinal overinvestments in symbolic figures. The problem arises when we are unable to see ourselves in this process. This notion of emancipatory fantasies aligns with my approach to the desire for social change. The key idea is the following:

> [...] there is something emancipatory in the structure of fantasy. Because fantasy depicts an excess that goes beyond what exists in the social order, it is a site from which the subject can access what necessarily remains invisible (and impossible) within the symbolic structure. Fantasy takes the subject beyond the rules that govern possible experience and thereby envisions the impossible. (McGowan, 2022, p. 193)

Based on my interpretation of the experience of the *estallido*, I concluded that the revolt reorganised the social bond in Chile but, to a significant extent, maintained the neoliberal libidinal economy in place. I derived this conclusion from the fact that the five fantasies identified in my analysis coalesced around a repudiation of negativity. Following McGowan's theorisation, this can be interpreted as a failure to include the subject in the fantasising. The main shared feature of all these fantasies is that, in none of them, was the subject able to perceive its own involvement in the imaginary narratives. Antagonism was constantly externalised; through their fantasies, subjects established an ideological distance from their own fantasmatic enjoyment. At least partially, the fantasmatic dimension of the revolt was not as emancipatory as the meanings in which the subjects were invested. Symbolically, Chile woke up but, on an imaginary level, the subjects could not see themselves awakening.

The way in which we forge unconscious attachments to emancipatory events is as important as the meanings emerging from these events. This is the dimension that my approach to the desire for social change brings to the fore, one that remains largely unattended in research. When the libidinal economy of the desire for social change is considered, emancipation appears less black and white; it becomes an internally divided process with its own dialectic between recognition and misrecognition. From a psychoanalytic perspective, this is the lesson of the *estallido.* What would including oneself in the fantasising look like? Simply put, although very difficult to bring into practice, it means making room for our lack of self-identity. Events like the Chilean revolt must deal with an excessive call, insofar as this is always the case with the Other. Such an excess is alienating but, at the same time, the reason why we can change. The potentially emancipatory role of fantasies comes from lessening of the psychic toll of alienation, not from rejecting it. Alienation is extremely difficult to endure, and fantasies often provide us with a getaway to avoid dealing with it. If fantasies can be emancipatory, they should allow us, at some level, to reduce the anxiety associated with our lack of self-identity. Which is nothing but another term for change.

References

Barthes, R. (1985). Of what use is an intellectual?. In *The Grain of the Voice. Interviews, 1962–1980*. Hill and Wang.

Canales, M. (2022). *La Pregunta de Octubre. Fundación, Apogeo y Crisis del Chile Neoliberal*. LOM Ediciones.

Castillo, A. (2019). *Asamblea de los Cuerpos*. Sangría Editora.

Chiesa, L. (2007). *Subjectivity and Otherness: A Philosophical Reading of Lacan*. The MIT Press.

Critchley, S. (2008). *Infinitely Demanding: Ethics of Commitment, Politics of Resistance*. Verso.

De Vivanco, L., & Johansson, M. (2021). Presentación. In L. de Vivanco & M. Johansson (Eds.), *Instantáneas en la Marcha. Repertorio de las Movilizaciones en Chile*. Ediciones Universidad Alberto Hurtado.

Dureuil, S. (2023). Psychoanalysis despite neoliberalism. *Psychoanalysis, Culture & Society, 28*(4), 534–550.

Edelman, L. (2007). *No Future: Queer Theory and the Death Drive*. Duke University Press.

Ffytche, M. (2019). Real fantasies: Reinserting the imaginary in the scene of social encounter. *Psychoanalysis, Culture & Society, 24*(4), 394–412.

Freud, S. (1981). Mourning and Melancholia. In *The Standard Edition of the Complete Psychological Works of Sigmund Freud, Vol. XIV (1914–1916)*. The Hogarth Press.

Glynos, J. (2011). On the ideological and political significance of fantasy in the organization of work. *Psychoanalysis, Culture & Society, 16*(4), 373–393.

Kapoor, I. (2020). *Confronting Desire. Psychoanalysis and International Development*. Cornell University Press.

Kapoor, I., Fridell, G., Sioh, M., & de Vries, P. (2023). *Global Libidinal Economy*. SUNY Press.

Kornbluh, A. (2019). *The Order of Forms. Realism, Formalism, and Social Space*. The University of Chicago Press.

Kornbluh, A. (2022). Solidarity words. *differences*, 33(2–3), 33–50.

Kristeva, J. (2025). *Intimate Revolt. The Powers and Limits of Psychoanalysis, Volume 2*. Columbia University Press.

Lacan, J. (1998). *The Seminar of Jacques Lacan, Book XI: The Four Fundamental Concepts of Psychoanalysis*. W. W. Norton & Company.

Lacan, J. (2007). *The Seminar of Jacques Lacan, Book XVII: The Other Side of Psychoanalysis*. W. W. Norton & Company.

Lacan, J. (2020). *The Seminar of Jacques Lacan, Book IV: The Object Relation*. Polity Press.

Laclau, E. (1990). *New Reflections on the Revolution of Our Time*. Verso.

López, M. (2021). Democracia e igualdad callejera: Acerca del octubre chileno. In L. de Vivanco & M. Johansson (Eds.), *Instantáneas en la Marcha. Repertorio de las Movilizaciones en Chile*. Ediciones Universidad Alberto Hurtado.

Mazzarella, W. (2017). *The Mana of Mass Society*. The University of Chicago Press.

McGowan, T. (2022). Mainstreaming fantasy: Politics without reserve. *differences, 33*(2–3), 177–197.

McGowan, T. (2025). *Pure Excess: Capitalism and the Commodity*. Columbia University Press.

McMillan, C. (2017). MakeAmericaGreatAgain: Ideological fantasy. *American exceptionalism and Donald Trump. Subjectivity, 10*(2), 204–222.

Neill, C. (2013). Breaking the text: An introduction to Lacanian discourse analysis. *Theory & Psychology, 23*(3), 334–350.

Proctor, H. (2024). *Burnout: The Emotional Experience of Political Defeat*. Verso.

Rancière, J. (2010). *La Noche de los Proletarios. Archivos del Sueño Obrero*. Tinta Limón.

Ronderos, S., & Glynos, J. (2022). Anti-populist fantasies: Interrogating Veja's discursive constructions, from Lula to Bolsonaro. *Critical Discourse Studies, 20*(6), 618–642.

Ruti, M. (2010). Life beyond fantasy: The rewriting of destiny in Lacanian theory. *Culture, Theory and Critique, 51*(1), 1–14.

Ruti, M. (2012). Reading Lacan as a social critic: What it means not to cede on one's desire. *Angelaki, 17*(1), 69–81.

Ruti, M. (2017). *The Ethics of Opting Out. Queer Theory's Defiant Subjects*. Columbia University Press.

Ruti, M. (2018). *Distillations: Theory, Ethics, Affect*. Bloomsbury Academic.

Safatle, V. (2022). Affects and politics. In S. Frosh, M. Vyrgioti, & J. Walsh (Eds.), *The Palgrave Handbook of Psychosocial Studies*. Palgrave Macmillan.

Sánchez, G., Valenzuela, F., & Sanfuentes, M. (2024). In pursuit of (post-)bureaucratic promises: Analyzing the logics of career self-management discourse at a privatized company. *Scandinavian Journal of Management, 40*(1), 101318.

Seitz, D., & Proudfoot, J. (2021). The psychic life of gentrification: Mapping desire and resentment in the gentrifying city. *Cultural Geographies, 28*(2), 213–219.

Uribe, M. (2020). *(18-O) Psicoanálisis de un Malestar: La Dignidad del Sujeto*. Descontexto Editores.

Vadolas, A. (2012). The bounced cheques of neoliberal fantasy: Anxiety in times of economic crisis. *Subjectivity, 5*(4), 355–375.

Woods, M. (2022). *On the Chilean Social Explosion*. Routledge.

Zupančič, A., & Terada, R. (2015). Sex, ontology, subjectivity: In conversation with Alenka Zupančič. *Psychoanalysis, Culture & Society, 20*(2), 192–206.

Appendix

The preparation for the fieldwork behind this book began with mapping postgraduate programmes in the humanities and social sciences in Chile. I retrieved the description, aims, and objectives of each programme from their websites. An initial screening allowed me to determine which ones aligned with a broadly defined critical approach. For instance, programmes that referred to the promotion of critical thinking, the development of critical tools, or made explicit links to knowledge production aimed at social change were included in my sample. For the observations, I shortlisted three programmes and used the others as a pool to contact potential interview participants. I then reached out to the directors of the three shortlisted programmes to present my study and request permission to observe some of their modules. All of them accepted. With the list of modules for the first semester of 2022 in hand, I proceeded to contact course convenors. Four academics agreed to let me observe their lessons, contingent on the students' consent. No student refused. In the end, I conducted observations in three modules across different universities.

Beginning this way not only allowed me to settle the most bureaucratic part of my fieldwork early on, but also gave me the opportunity to connect with scholars and students for interviews. With the exception

G. Sánchez, *A Rebel Unconscious*, Studies in the Psychosocial,
https://doi.org/10.1007/978-3-032-12275-9

Table 1 Interviews summary

Participants	Pseudonym	Gender	Age	Background
Scholars	Verónica*	Female	50	Philosophy
	Isabel	Female	47	Education
	Cristina	Female	47	History
	Sofía*	Female	39	Sociology
	Carlos	Male	44	Philosophy
	Rodrigo	Male	42	Cultural Studies
	Ramón*	Male	44	Philosophy
PhD researchers	Carmen	Female	31	Sociology
	María	Female	35	Education
	Daniela	Female	31	Education
	Catalina	Female	32	Communication
	Lorena	Female	43	Psychology
	Arturo	Male	29	Cultural Studies
	Nicolás	Male	38	Aesthetics

of a handful of academics who declined—either because their workload made it impossible or because they were on sabbatical—the vast majority of those I contacted accepted my invitation or pointed me to colleagues who might be interested. My initial plan was to interview five scholars and five postgraduate students three times each, a strategy inspired by psychoanalytic designs. Very quickly, however, it became clear that this was unrealistic. While many expressed interest in the study, they declined participation once they learned how time-consuming the design would be. I therefore reduced the number of interviews per participant and broadened the sample instead. In the end, I interviewed seven scholars and seven postgraduate students, each twice. Table 1 summarises the participants in my study. Asterisks next to some pseudonyms indicate individuals who also convened the modules I observed. To safeguard anonymity, I chose not to disclose the module titles. In total, I observed 15 lessons, amounting to 45 hours of classroom activity.

Even after revising my design and expectations, I still had to make further adjustments, as I produced more empirical material than I could reasonably handle on my own. Once my fieldwork was complete, I went back to the UK and fully transcribed the first set of fourteen interviews, which came to 148 pages (or 92,016 words), alongside two mid-size notebooks of observations and a personal notebook with reflections written after each interview. If this picture is not vivid enough, the sheer volume of this corpus felt like a sea without a coastline. The richness of the material was as impressive as it was intimidating. I therefore decided to focus my analysis on the first fourteen interviews, while listening to the other fourteen and drawing on them for context or clarification.

In my interpretation, I did not follow a ready-made template. After transcribing the interviews, I read through all the material several times simply to familiarise myself with it. Only once this process was complete did I begin to identify the themes around which participants' associations clustered. I did not use any data analysis software—only Excel, to list the themes I noted down. I experimented with several ways of organising these themes in order to build a narrative structure for the analysis. After months of work (and discarding a few failed attempts), I realised that, despite the dispersion of the material, many themes could be grouped into two general activities: seeing and writing. This insight allowed me to bring the *estallido* into dialogue with a specific practice, making the empirical corpus more manageable. With this structure in mind, I returned to the material and began identifying the signifiers that organised these practices. I insisted on sitting with those signifiers repeatedly, trusting that this insistence would reveal their materiality—that point at which their autonomy becomes evident. It was through this process that I reconstructed the five fantasies presented in this book.

Index

G. Sánchez, *A Rebel Unconscious*, Studies in the Psychosocial, https://doi.org/10.1007/978-3-032-12275-9